Finding
Purpose
in the
Pause

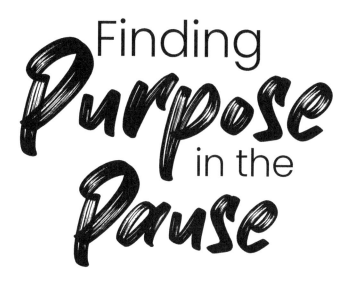

Finding Purpose in the Pause

Your Guide to Thriving in Menopause and Beyond

Carol Covino

ISBN: 979-8-88759-530-6 (paperback)
ISBN: 979-8-88759-531-3 (ebook)

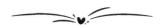

I dedicate this book to my family—my husband, Mike; my daughters, Francesca and Sophia; and my son, Tony. Thank you for encouraging me to follow my heart and inspiring me to grow. I love you all so much.

With a woman's life expectancy at eighty-four years, it is reasonable to expect that she will not only live thirty to forty years beyond menopause, but be vibrant, sharp, and influential as well. The menopause you will experience is not your mother's (or grandmother's) menopause.

—Christiane Northrup,
The Wisdom of Menopause: Creating Physical and Emotional Health During the Change

Contents

Preface

A Woman I Knew

There was a woman I knew. As a little girl growing up in the turbulent 1960s, she lived in a hundred-year-old three-bedroom home with one bathroom and no shower in southern California. The house had almost burned to the ground under its original owner and still had the stale, stank odor of smoke. There were four bedrooms if you count the makeshift sunroom room that served as her older brothers' bedroom and only one bathroom with an old, moldy tub.

The girl slept in a dark bedroom with no windows. Her parents did the best they could, but both had their own dragons to slay. Her father came from poverty and domestic abuse. He grew up in a bedroom above their church with his mother and sister during the Great Depression. He later joined the Army after Pearl Harbor in December of 1941, where he became trained as an expert sniper and machine gunner. He was part of the original troops that touched down in Normandy on D-day in 1944. After the war, he suffered what was then referred to as "battle shock" and "combat fatigue." We now call it post-traumatic stress disorder (PTSD).

From the age of four, she remembers hearing stories of his flashbacks and witnessing his ongoing nightmares and hypervigilance. In the midst of his flashbacks, he had once jumped out of a two-story window, breaking his leg. Another time, he attempted to jump out of a moving vehicle when he heard a car backfire. The girl awoke one night to her mother's frightened pleas. She wandered into her parents' bedroom to see her father choking her mother. The girl called out loudly, waking her father from his nightmare. She would later learn this was a regular occurrence when her father had nightmares.

The girl would watch her father lapse into long, dark silences where he would seem to go away to someplace very far and sad. She watched as he took 14 Excedrin a day to ease his constant crippling headaches. Decades later he would ask her to sneak those Excedrin into his hospital room. The girl understood she wasn't to ask any questions of her father. She would just sit by his side until the darkness passed. Her mother would simply whisper, "It's because of the war."

Her father slept with his clothes on and a gun nearby in case he would need to fight or flee with his family in the night. There was constant tension, arguments, and anger in her home. She would lie in her small twin bed in the room with no windows. She was certain there were ghosts in the old, creaky home, so she often fought sleep, thinking she would not be safe if she drifted off. There were fights between her parents and fights between her older brother and her father.

Her brother was one of four children from her mother's first marriage to an abusive man with a gambling addiction. They lived in extreme poverty and were frequently evicted from their rental homes. Her mother had remarried a year after fleeing Oklahoma with her two young sons. She landed in an apartment in southern California. It was there she met the girl's father who was carrying out empty whiskey bottles to the trash dumpster. They were married in less than a year. Her mother did not marry out of love. She married out of survival. She needed a provider for her sons. She naively believed that this quiet, war-torn veteran would be the gentle husband she desperately needed.

A year later she gave birth to the girl. The girl's father had a strong, fearful, and possessive attachment to his daughter. Nothing mattered except her. From there, the turmoil and abuse began. The girl was torn. She loved this man she called her father, but she saw that his quiet exterior hid dark moods and an inward rage. The girl would lie in her room with no windows, in fear. She would listen to the angry voices and was afraid of what her father would do. She was afraid of the anger and resentment she saw in her older brothers. She was afraid to go to sleep, thinking something terrible would happen in the night.

As the girl entered first grade, her fears and anxiety followed her into the schoolroom. She would stare out the window, imagining a fairytale life to escape the turmoil inside her body. As a consequence, she didn't learn to read. It was 1967 and childhood trauma was not something recognized by the educational system. You conformed, or you were punished and pushed aside.

After testing, the girl was placed in a program for the "slow kids." She was labeled "mentally retarded" (as it was called in the 1960s). This was when a beautiful, young teacher saved the girl. The teacher sat down with the child and patiently taught her to read and write. The girl would later read at a twelfth-grade high school level when she was only in the fifth grade and a college level by the time she reached the seventh grade. Despite these accomplishments, the damage was done. The girl had labeled herself "stupid," a label that would stick for decades.

When the girl was 11, something which reinforced her fears happened. Her father always slept fully clothed with a gun nearby. One night a drunken neighbor began aimlessly shooting a gun from his balcony. As the shots rang out in the small neighborhood, the girl was frozen in her bed. Then her father burst through the door. He threw her down on the floor and told her not to move. There was a gun in his hand. The girl watched in terror as he made his way down the hall. She saw his face and knew he intended to kill the man shooting. The police arrived before this could happen, and the crazed neighbor was taken away. Nighttime was, indeed, a time of terror.

The girl became a young teen eager for new experiences, yet her father's possessiveness prevented her from having many of these rites of passage. There was no dating, and she did not have the chance to be with friends until her parents separated for the first time. There would be a reunion between them after a year. However, ultimately the marriage would end.

When the girl turned 21, she became involved in an abusive relationship. She had little experience with men and found herself whisked into what appeared to be a storybook romance. "Happily ever after" quickly turned into verbal and physical abuse that left her feeling a shadow of herself. She could have left. Yet, she felt she didn't deserve anything better. Every time he told her she was stupid and worthless, it only reinforced what she already believed to be true.

Eventually she found the courage to leave. She married a man who treated her well and made her feel safe (at least for a time). They wanted a family. However, this "happily ever after" scenario would slip away from the woman once again. She suffered for ten years through several miscarriages and surgeries.

At age 34, she miscarried twins and this sent her spiraling into depression. A year later the couple made the decision to adopt. She and her husband adopted the first of three beautiful children from China. Her childhood and the past abuse seemed far away and almost like something that had happened to someone else. Again, she felt safe and fulfilled for a time.

In her mid-forties, the woman decided one day she would run a marathon. She trained for 12 weeks to accomplish the task and ran her first race. She took first place in the master's category, top five overall, and qualified for the Boston Marathon. From that point forward, she became obsessed with running.

She would drive her three young, school-age children, two years apart in age, from one activity to the next. She was running 75 to 100 miles per week to train and regularly attending spin classes and fitness bootcamps. She used exercise as a way to exhaust herself in hopes of a good night's sleep. She used exercise to clear her mind. She used exercise to numb out. She used exercise so she could eat whatever she wanted.

As she moved through her forties, sleep became even more difficult. By the time she was 48, she wasn't sleeping more than three hours per night. In the morning, she could barely drag herself out of bed. Despite all the exercise, she was flabby and had a pooch in her lower belly. She felt unattractive and frumpy.

If a few pounds crept on, she doubled down on her exercise and slashed calories. She drank diet Cokes and ate refined carbs. Her idea of protein was a grilled cheese or peanut-butter-and-jelly sandwich. The extreme exercise simply made things worse.

One morning as she stepped down on the cold tile floor and tried to make her way to the coffee pot, she felt extreme pain in both feet. It was as if she were stepping down on sharp crystals. As she moved awkwardly down the hall to wake the children for school, the pain gradually dissipated. She decided it was just due to age and arthritis from running.

She then began to suffer profound fatigue. Every day she had to lie down and nap for an hour before the school bus arrived with her young son. At the same time, she was experiencing sharp debilitating pain in her stomach, which would occur suddenly and leave her doubled up in pain. After a trip to the ER and numerous tests, including a colonoscopy, she was diagnosed with IBS (irritable bowel syndrome). She was prescribed pain medication to control the attacks and left to deal with the unpredictable symptoms.

What about that bone-crushing fatigue and excruciating pain in her feet? After years of doctors' visits and feeling as if she had lost her mind, her podiatrist noticed an unusual pattern of joint damage in both feet. One was a mirror image of the other. He brought up the images on a screen and explained this was not the pattern of osteoarthritis. Rather it was a sign of a much more serious autoimmune condition called rheumatoid arthritis (RA), an autoimmune condition that attacks the joints and even organs such as the heart and lungs.

It would take eight months and the emergence of unexplained kidney problems for the final diagnosis. As she sat in the nephrologist's office, he handed her the grim news. Every inflammation marker in her lab report was elevated high above the norm. She was sent to a rheumatologist who diagnosed her with an autoimmune disease, rheumatoid arthritis.

What she didn't know at the time was that her past lifestyle habits along with unresolved trauma had ignited the firestorm of inflammation responsible for IBS and RA. As she struggled with the joint and stomach pain, her body betrayed her even further with sudden lightening hot flashes and drenching night sweats. Despite cold winter nights where temperatures would dip down into the twenties, she would throw open every bedroom window. She would awake drenched and shaking from the cold.

She no longer enjoyed sex and often avoided her husband's attempts to be intimate. She wondered if that part of her life was over. She could not share these feelings with anyone. At this point, her mother had passed away from heart failure. Even if she were still living, menopause was a topic that was off limits. Perimenopause was a complete mystery. The media wasn't discussing midlife women, and they certainly weren't talking about menopause. The doctors weren't having conversations with their older female patients. The culture was entirely fixated on youth. There was no room for a woman with hormonal imbalance, night sweats, and hot flashes.

As she looked in the mirror, she no longer recognized the woman looking back at her. This woman was thin but her legs were flabby and her glutes were flat. When she turned to the side, that belly pooch was becoming more prominent. New lines and wrinkles on her face seemed to be appearing daily. She felt a sense of shame that her own body had betrayed her.

This woman was me. That little girl was me. The combination of over-exercising, stress, lack of sleep, a poor diet, and a traumatic past wreaked havoc. My lifestyle was no longer working. I needed help. I reached out to a personal trainer who started me on a weight training plan. Slowly, I saw muscle tone appear in my shoulders and legs. Under his guidance I became a group fitness instructor and later a personal trainer.

Despite my growing knowledge of exercise, there was something missing. I continued to do excessive amounts of cardio and to eat a diet that consisted of too many sweets, poor carbohydrate choices, and unhealthy fats. It was at this time that a friend did a bikini bodybuilding show. I was fascinated as I watched her body transform. Gone was the excess body fat and in its place beautiful muscle tone. As I watched her grace the stage, I made a decision. I wanted that body.

I questioned my friend and determined that diet was the key and, in particular, protein was the solution. I didn't know how much or even what sources of protein to eat. To me protein was cheese and peanut butter with an occasional hamburger or chicken breast.

I sought the advice of my personal trainer who encouraged me to give up running and change my diet. I worked to prepare for my first competition. After several months, I hit the stage at a skinny 110 pounds. I had increased muscle tone and eliminated the belly fat, but I still did not have the body I desired.

In frustration, I spent hours scouring the web for bikini competitors close to my age who could help me. I only found one, and she lived out of state and was not taking clients. Eventually, I ran across the Facebook page of an Albuquerque woman in her early thirties who was a professional bodybuilding champion. She was tall, muscular, and beautiful with the legs I wanted.

I contacted her and began working with her to prepare for my second bikini show. This was when my body began to change. The running was replaced with weightlifting and the StairMaster. I now knew what protein sources to eat and how much. I was weighing and measuring my food. Pasta was replaced with sweet potatoes and vegetables. Instead of diet Cokes, I drank a gallon of water each day. Gone were the late-night cookies and bowls of chocolate chip mint ice cream.

My coach introduced me to a nurse practitioner who specializes in hormone replacement therapy (HRT) for women. I was terrified of using hormones. Would they cause cancer? However, I was desperate to control the hot flashes, low libido, and lack of sleep. She started me on a bio-identical estrogen and progesterone cream as well as a testosterone cream. The HRT combined with the changes in my exercise and nutrition made a difference. The night sweats and crazy hot flashes disappeared, my sleep improved, and my sexual desire returned. This was when I knew I was on the right track. This marked the beginning of my quest and mission to help other midlife women look and feel better than they could ever imagine.

I went from being a burned-out marathon runner to becoming a top three figure bodybuilding champion on the national stage. In addition to group fitness and personal training, I became a certified yoga instructor and fitness nutritionist. I opened my own exercise studio where I taught classes and trained women in weightlifting and nutrition. Today I focus exclusively on virtually coaching women over 40 and hosting my podcast, *Forever Fit with Carol Covino*.

Yet, it would not be until age 54 that I realized I needed to address the past trauma. It had seeped into my marriage and was preventing me from truly living my purpose. With the help of a therapist who specializes in women's trauma, I began to unlock the reasons I had become sick with autoimmune. I stopped using exercise to numb out. I unpacked areas of my life that had left me broken. I learned coping skills for triggers.

This is now my passion, my life's work, and why I wrote this book.

Chapter 1

Menopause Is Natural. Suffering Is Optional

I first met Patricia at the local gym. I was finishing up a set of squats when she approached me. Patricia explained that she had heard my latest podcast on balancing hormones for weight loss and was interested in working with me. She was in her late forties and experiencing many common perimenopausal symptoms, such as fatigue, poor sleep, and weight gain in her midsection.

"These extra pounds make me feel oldI and tired," she said in a low, dejected tone. "I run on the treadmill most days and barely eat anything. The weight won't come off, and I can't stand how big my stomach looks."

Perimenopause is the five to seven years leading into menopause where women can experience fluctuations in estrogen and progesterone and problems handling the effects of stress. As a widow with two teen boys and working a demanding job in healthcare, Patricia was no stranger to stress.

Under my guidance, Patricia reduced refined foods and increased protein. She replaced running with walking and began lifting weights for the first time in her life. She eliminated *nighttime cardio sessions and planned her workouts earlier in the day to help with sleep. In three months, Patricia lost 15 pounds, five inches off her waist, and four inches from her hips. She took her waist-to-hip ratio from high risk for diabetes and heart disease down to a low risk. More importantly, she told me she loved her body, and her entire life had changed for the better.*

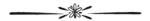

As women navigate through their forties and fifties into the second half of life, they face unique challenges. Hormones begin to shift. They may experience weight gain, loss of muscle tone, fatigue, brain fog, anxiety, lack of sleep, loss of libido, and hot flashes. A woman may not feel like herself anymore. She can experience a sense of loss. It can seem as if life isn't all it should be.

As given in my story in this book's preface, I suffered needlessly through the transition into menopause. Looking back, I'm not sure how I made it through to the other side. Now I want to lift the veil of shame and unlock the ways you can make this the most beautiful and fulfilling time of your life.

This brings us to the journey you and I are about to take right now. This is your opportunity to have a transformative experience that will give you the power to change both your body and your life. I believe there are several key pillars a woman must have before she can transition well through midlife and into this second half of life—nutrition, the right kind of exercise, sleep, and the management of stress and past trauma. Therefore, through this book, together we will boost your metabolism, increase your hormonal health, boost your energy, clear the brain fog, build lean muscle tone, and decrease body fat.

Every woman, despite sharing common experiences, has her own unique metabolism and makeup based on age, stage of life, and health needs. I'll be helping you find your distinct "bio-individuality." Chapter by chapter, I will be educating you on the lifestyle habits that affect your hormones.

By the time I reached my late forties, it became apparent that the things I had done for the past 25 years were no longer serving me. At the time, no one was talking about menopause. The very word was associated with secrecy, loss, and shame. Because I didn't understand the changes in my body, I experienced health problems, burnout, and a collision with past trauma that was exasperated by the physical symptoms. Through my bodybuilding transformation, I learned the power of nutrition and the right type of exercise.

Over the past decade, I have guided over a thousand women to transformation. I created the Fit and Fierce coaching program and the *Forever Fit with Carol Covino* podcast for women over 40. Now I will be giving you the exact method I use to help women maintain a healthy weight and body fat percentage, build muscle, increase bone strength, and naturally balance hormones. This is not a weight loss program. This is a lifestyle.

Here are some comments from women who participated in my Fit and Fierce coaching program:

- From Annette: *I couldn't settle on one "greatest benefit" in this program. There were so many. I learned how to eat, my hormones are balanced, my body changed shape, and pounds and inches were lost. And my hubby is so excited with his own post heart attack progress. The program gave me a jumpstart on cooking and guiding his nutrition.*
- From Katrina: *I lost 10 pounds! I have a better understanding of what my caloric intake should be as*

well as my protein, carbs, and fats. I feel like I now have the knowledge needed to adjust my own macros.

- From Naomi: *I can see my body reshaping. I feel more in control of my health instead of feeling like I'm in a downhill motion.*
- From Melanie: *I'm down 10 pounds since I started the program, but 16 pounds since I started following Carol. I lost three inches off my waist and five inches from my hips. The macros were very liberating for me, and I did not feel restricted.*
- From Georgia: *I learned what and how to eat. I lost six pounds and three inches. I reshaped my body and got my hormones in check. So many benefits!*

The Three Phases

The program that these women followed so successfully—as well as the content of this book—is based on the following three phases:

Phase 1—Hormones

First, you will learn which hormones are affecting your metabolism and what nutrition choices will support hormone health to help you lose body fat, build lean muscle growth, and create metabolic flexibility.

Phase 2—Building Muscle

Second, you will learn how to exercise to build muscle and reshape your body in perimenopause, menopause, and beyond. I will teach you the exercise mistakes to avoid that accelerate aging and cause you to hold on to body fat.

Phase 3—Self-Care

Third, we will address the lifestyle habits that support hormone balance, including sleep, stress, and supplementation. Self-care is critical past age 40 when our body goes through hormonal fluctuations and shifts as we move toward menopause. Self-care is more than a day at the spa. It's everything from quality sleep to dealing with stress and past trauma.

I understand where you are and what it's like to feel the shifts and changes in your body. I too struggled with belly fat, food cravings, lack of sleep, hot flashes, anxiety, depression, and exhaustion. I will never forget what it was like to feel that loss of hope and despair. Because of this, I can support you and help you regain the vitality and energy you thought was lost. Let this book be life-changing for you, something you refer back to time and time again to help you not only achieve results but sustain them. You no longer have to suffer with stubborn weight gain, body fat, brain fog, depression, and fatigue.

Are you ready for the second half of life and for both a transformation of the body and the mind? Let's get started!

Chapter 2

What's Going On With My Hormones?

Tammy came to me at age 48, exhausted and frustrated with her weight gain. She had tried numerous diet programs that reduced calories and increased cardio with little to no change. Tammy was in the throes of perimenopause, those pivotal years leading into menopause. She was so unhappy with her body that she was embarrassed to wear shorts and sleeveless tops because of her legs and arms. She felt defeated when she caught sight of her reflection in the shop windows.

Tammy's cravings were high and sleep was low. She felt the stress in every part of her body. Anxiety and brain fog were regular occurrences. We increased her lean protein intake, brought her dietary fats and carbohydrates in balance, reduced her cardio, introduced strength training, and established a nighttime routine to help with sleep. In addition, she developed a stress management plan to help her deal with the demands of work. She lost 30 pounds and over eight inches. Today she wears short skirts and sleeveless tops and even did a photo shoot to celebrate her body. She's energetic and confident.

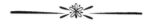

Perhaps you feel like Tammy once felt. You've exercised and reduced calories, lost a few pounds, only to gain it back and more. Your sleep is poor and energy is low. You just don't feel like yourself anymore, and your body is slowly changing. The old method of "eat less and exercise more" no longer works.

The truth is—it never worked. You were just more resilient in your twenties and thirties. You had the protection of some key hormones. As those hormones shift and fluctuate, so does your body. We have to change the lifestyle habits that affect the hormones that affect fat loss. It's not about calories. It's about hormones and the quality of the food we eat.

Something happens as you transition from your forties into menopause. It becomes easier to gain weight. Your body takes on a different shape as weight starts to redistribute to the midsection. Your cravings are stronger. Mood swings and brain fog begin to emerge. Energy is low. It becomes more difficult to deal with stress. You feel the signs of aging.

I get it. You're not alone. I've experienced this myself, and I've seen these symptoms in the women who come to me for help. I want to encourage you—it's never too late, and you're never too old. I did not prioritize my health until I was 50 years old, yet I have been able to transform my body and my mind.

Let's take a look at some of the key hormones and how nutrition and lifestyle choices affect those hormones. The hormones we'll look at are cortisol, insulin, leptin, ghrelin, glucagon, estrogen, progesterone, testosterone, DHEA, thyroid hormones, and growth hormone. We'll also look into testing to determine hormone imbalances.

Cortisol—The Stress Hormone

Cortisol provides energy in times of acute stress. It's known as your "fight, flight, or freeze hormone." This is the hormone responsible for the action you need to take to survive threats. Think of fleeing a lion.

When you're stressed out, your body perceives it is under attack. The sympathetic nervous system (SNS) sends a signal to the adrenal glands to pump the hormone epinephrine (adrenaline) into the bloodstream. Blood is then directed to the heart, muscles, and organs. Your blood pressure and pulse increase, and your breathing becomes rapid.

The hypothalamus releases corticotropin-releasing hormone (CRH) that goes to the adrenal glands and prompts them to put out cortisol. Cortisol releases blood sugar to give you the energy and strength you need to defend yourself. It also increases blood pressure, so you can have enough oxygen and nutrients in your body.

Once the threat is gone, cortisol levels typically fall. The parasympathetic nervous (PNS) takes over and calms your body.

The problem lies with the chronic stress we encounter daily in our present-day society. Stress now takes the form of traffic, work deadlines, a nasty text, marital problems, financial difficulties, and even the grim news headlines that greet us each morning. In fact, stress seems to be everywhere. Many people are living life in a perpetual state of fight or flight because of chronic stress. Their sympathetic nervous system is continually activated.

Another aspect of the body's stress response is that a part of the brain called the amygdala overrides the prefrontal cortex, which is the reasoning and thinking side of the brain. This overriding, in turn, affects our ability to be rational and to make wise decisions, which, in turn, keeps us in a stressed state or perhaps even increases the stress levels we're experiencing.

Cortisol is a vital part of our health, and we can't live without it. For example, cortisol:

- Protects cardiovascular health
- Regulates appetite
- Controls cravings
- Acts as an anti-inflammatory if you are injured, have arthritis, or suffer with allergies
- Increases concentration, awareness, mood, and cognitive function
- Allows your muscles to properly respond to exercise
- Stimulates the immune system

However, cortisol becomes an issue when we are chronically stressed. When the body becomes flooded with cortisol, it interferes with other hormones, including insulin, estrogen, progesterone, and testosterone. If we remain in a state of stress, the sympathetic nervous system (SNS) becomes overactive, resulting in metabolic problems that then might lead to chronic inflammation, high insulin, low immunity, and other health problems.

In order to comprehend the effects of the "fight or flight" response on the body, we need to have an understanding of the SNS. The sympathetic nervous system is part of the autonomic nervous system. It's a group of nerves primarily located just outside the spinal cord that is controlled by the hypothalamus of the brain. It is activated by danger or stress and affects your eyes, heart, lungs, and digestive tract. The SNS slows down the digestive process, so you can utilize that energy to respond to threats. Also, your body releases an influx of glucose (sugar) into the bloodstream for a quick energy boost. Blood sugar dysregulation is associated with metabolic issues. Thus, the strain of ongoing stress and anxiety on your sympathetic nervous system can lead to obesity and metabolic dysfunction.

Cortisol can cause weight gain and the storage of visceral body fat. This is the fat that is under the white fat in your midsection and surrounds vital internal organs to protect them. Too much visceral fat is dangerous and puts you at a greater risk of heart attack, stroke, and type 2 diabetes. Cortisol speeds up the accumulation of body fat by sending triglycerides from storage to the visceral fat cells. The fat cells have enzymes containing even more cortisol.

Triglycerides are attracted to visceral fat because we have a multitude of receptors there. In fact, we have four times more cortisol receptors in visceral belly fat than in subcutaneous fat (the fat just below the skin). This results in what is called the "cortisol belly"—fat around the waistline from too much stress.

High blood sugar causes higher cortisol that results in the storage of visceral fat. Excess cortisol causes the body to break down protein reserves into glucose to be used as fuel and stored as fat. Cortisol also moves fat stores from elsewhere in the body to visceral body fat.

Cortisol also increases your appetite and cravings for carbohydrates and sugar. A study at the University of California revealed in the lab that premenopausal women who had higher cortisol during and after stressful events ate more foods high in fat and sugar.

There are several lifestyle habits that affect cortisol levels, including lack of sleep, over-exercising, under-eating, and perceived daily stress. Prioritizing sleep, eating quality food, and having a stress management plan will help to reduce and stabilize cortisol levels.

Insulin

Insulin is secreted by the pancreas and is our key metabolic hormone. It plays a big role in blood-sugar levels (glucose), growth and repair of cells, weight control, brain function, and metabolism.

After you eat, your digestive system breaks down your food and extracts the nutrients, so they can be absorbed by the cells and tissues of the body. Carbohydrates are broken down into glucose (sugar) that is absorbed into your bloodstream. The glucose temporarily rises after eating. Your pancreas releases insulin. Insulin moves the glucose to the cells. The higher the blood glucose, the more insulin your pancreas releases.

Insulin shuttles glucose to your cells for energy and attaches to insulin receptors on cells throughout the body. It signals the cells to let the glucose in. This is key to metabolic flexibility. This means your body can access fuel from fat, glucose, or glycogen (stored glucose) for energy. Once the glucose enters your cells, blood sugar levels should go back to normal.

When you eat food, glucose rises, and insulin is secreted to bring those blood sugar levels down. When you don't need glucose for energy, your body stores it in the liver and muscles as glycogen. Glycogen is used by the body when you need a quick burst of energy. Glycogen can be broken down into glucose and used as fuel.

Once the glycogen stores reach their limit, the excess is converted to a fat called triglycerides. Triglycerides circulate in the bloodstream to increase energy or are stored in your fat tissue. If you eat more carbohydrates than your body can store, it will deposit them into the fat cells. Insulin regulates this process by inhibiting the breakdown of fat for energy (lipolysis). Over time, this can cause fat gain.

When you have elevated insulin from eating too many refined carbohydrates and too much sugar, you can potentially develop insulin resistance. This is where the cells become less receptive to insulin. The receptors no longer open up to allow the hormone to move glucose from the bloodstream into the cells. Picture the cell becoming overwhelmed with insulin and telling it to go away.

Insulin resistance can increase hot flashes and night sweats and lead to type 2 diabetes, certain cancers, heart disease, and other chronic illnesses. When insulin combines with cortisol, they can gang up on you to create havoc. Insulin and cortisol levels both increase under stress. Cortisol prepares your body to deal with stress by increasing blood sugar to provide energy for your muscles. It also slows down insulin production to prevent glucose from being stored so that glucose can be immediately used. If cortisol is continually elevated, the body can remain insulin resistant.

When someone has insulin imbalance, they are not metabolically flexible. This means that the body cannot switch between burning fat for fuel and burning carbohydrates (sugar) for fuel. When you are a carb (sugar or glucose) burner, your body has no reason to reach for fat as fuel. Your body is running on carbohydrates. You become caught in a vicious cycle. The more carbs you eat, the higher the blood glucose goes, requiring more insulin to return those levels to normal. Insulin spikes cause the sugar (glucose) burner to hold on to body fat. High body fat makes you less likely to respond to insulin and can lead to insulin resistance. In turn, insulin resistance causes inflammation, heart disease, and type 2 diabetes. Research has shown that people who have prediabetes or type 2 diabetes are metabolically inflexible.

However, this can potentially be reversed with nutrition and lifestyle changes.

In women, insulin imbalance can have many consequences, included among them are the following:

- Uncontrollable cravings for carbohydrates and sugar. The brain sends signals to the hypothalamus when blood sugar drops, which result in very strong cravings.
- Estrogen dominance caused by excess estrogen, which can, in turn, cause PMS (premenstrual syndrome), ovarian cysts, heavy periods, endometriosis, and benign breast disease.
- Fluid retention caused by the effect of high insulin on your kidneys. The kidneys then hold on to salt and water.
- An imbalance in dopamine and serotonin, which are responsible for hunger cues (among other things).
- A hormonal disorder called polycystic ovary syndrome (PCOS) can potentially be triggered by excess insulin, inflammation, heredity, and an excess of male hormones. Symptoms include prolonged periods, cysts in the ovaries, problems conceiving, and infrequent periods.

Lifestyle habits that negatively affect insulin include frequent snacking, consuming ultra-refined carbohydrates and sugar, and not enough movement or exercise. Intermittent fasting—the practice of alternating periods of fasting (not eating) with specific time windows where food is consumed—can help by lowering insulin levels, thus allowing you to use up stored sugar and to use fat as fuel. One 2018 study found that intermittent fasting reversed insulin resistance and allowed patients to eventually wean off insulin therapy. They also lost weight and reduced their waist circumference. We will be diving deeper into the benefits of intermittent fasting and how to incorporate it as a lifestyle in chapter 4.

The Hunger Hormones

Leptin

Leptin, known as the satiety hormone, was first discovered by scientists in 1994. This hormone plays a role in reducing hunger and is found in the white fat cells as well as brown fat tissue, ovaries, the lower part of your stomach, and in the muscle.

Leptin helps you maintain your weight by causing you to feel full and satisfied after a meal. However, it is also more than just a hunger hormone. Leptin also does the following:

- Regulates immunity
- Burns triglycerides as fuel (blood fats)
- Determines fat storage
- Takes part in the formation of bone
- Controls blood pressure and heart rate
- Regulates inflammation and wound healing
- Helps create new blood vessels and blood cells
- Controls thyroid function

In some individuals, the feeling of being full does not occur. Their brain does not detect leptin. They crave more food and have insatiable cravings for refined and sugary carbohydrates. This is a hormonal imbalance called leptin resistance.

With leptin resistance, a cycle occurs where the more you eat, the more you gain fat, and the less sensitive your body becomes to leptin. Leptin resistance can be the cause of weight gain and can possibly affect your thyroid, which, in turn, can slow your metabolism. Leptin resistance can also elevate blood pressure and contribute to mood disorders.

Leptin resistance is caused by obesity, a diet high in addictive, inflammatory ultra-processed food, poor sleep, continually high insulin levels, and lack of exercise.

Lifestyle habits that negatively affect leptin are sleep deficiency and restrictive low-calorie diets. Dieting should not be a hobby.

Ghrelin

Ghrelin is the hunger hormone that sends you the signal to eat when it's been too long between meals. It stimulates your appetite, causing you to eat more food and to store fat. Ghrelin is primarily produced and released by your stomach and is regulated by the parasympathetic nervous system (PNS). Ghrelin stimulates hunger, and you eat a meal in response. Then the PNS sends a message to the digestive system to rest and digest the food. Ghrelin then subsides.

Ghrelin also causes the release of growth hormone to break down fat tissue and promote muscle growth. In addition, ghrelin controls the release of insulin and protects the cardiovascular system.

When you go on a diet to lose weight, ghrelin levels rise. The longer you restrict calories, the higher your levels will be.

Ghrelin works in conjunction with leptin. However, any upset in the balance of the two hormones causes increased appetite, overeating, cravings for sweets and carbs, and a slower metabolism.

Lifestyle habits negatively affecting ghrelin are sleep deficiency, extended low-calorie diets, and stress.

Glucagon

Glucagon is the fat-releasing hormone secreted by the pancreas. It works with insulin to regulate and stabilize blood glucose (sugar) levels by preventing them from falling too low. It converts stored carbohydrates in the liver to glucose. When your brain receives the message that your body needs food, it secretes glucagon.

While insulin is a fat-storing hormone, Glucagon is a fat-burning hormone. When glucose (sugar) is too low, glucagon stimulates the breakdown of fat, so your body can use it for ongoing energy.

Glucagon primarily works on the liver to prevent blood glucose from falling too low. It converts glycogen (stored carbohydrates) to glucose to enter the bloodstream for fuel. It stimulates the production of glucose from amino acids, and it decreases glucose usage by the liver.

Imbalance of glucagon is rare. However, if your blood glucose levels frequently and drastically rise and fall, your body may have abnormal glucagon levels. Signs are low blood sugar, dizziness, fatigue, lightheadedness, and confusion.

One lifestyle habit that can help with glucagon levels and fat burning is intermittent fasting. When intermittent fasting, glucagon then steps in to stabilize blood sugar levels to prevent them from becoming too low. The fat-burning effects can be further stimulated by increasing protein and decreasing carbohydrates during the feeding window. This increases glucagon, preventing your body from producing too much insulin and keeping blood sugar at stable levels. This can result in less fat storage and more fat burning.

Estrogen

Estrogen refers to three female hormones. Estradiol (E2) is the form we have in our reproductive years and is the most powerful one. It's secreted from the ovaries and is responsible for increasing sex drive and moisturizing body tissues. Levels begin to fluctuate in perimenopause and decline significantly in menopause.

Estriol (E3) makes up about 10 percent of our estrogen but is the form that is most abundant in pregnancy where it is produced by the placenta.

Estrone (E1) is the form that dominates during menopause. It's weaker than estradiol and accounts for about 10 percent of total estrogen. It is created by the fat cells, adrenal glands, and the ovaries.

When estrogen is balanced, it results in soft skin and positively affects memory. It prevents inflammation, helps to regulate weight, and protects against cardiovascular disease. Much of midlife weight gain can be due to shifts in estrogen levels. Combined with a loss in muscle and a greater tendency to insulin resistance, this causes many women to struggle with their weight as they get older.

Progesterone

Progesterone is a hormone that is made in the ovaries up until menopause. After menopause, it is produced by the adrenal glands. Progesterone balances estrogen, helps regulate sleep and body temperature, helps with bone formation, maintains stable blood sugar levels, supports the thyroid, relaxes the gut muscles so you can break down nutrients, and is a natural diuretic.

Progesterone stimulates gamma-aminobutyric acid (GABA), allowing you to feel calmer, less anxious and irritable, and less prone to mood swings. It naturally declines when ovulation becomes less frequent in perimenopause and when you reach menopause. Signs of low progesterone are anxiety, sleep disturbances, night sweats, hot flashes, migraines, weight gain, shorter menstrual cycles, breast tenderness, and PMS.

Intermittent fasting can help support and balance progesterone levels. However, if you are still having a monthly period, you should not fast five to seven days before your menstruation. Otherwise, you could deplete progesterone.

Estrogen and Progesterone Imbalance

An imbalance between estrogen and progesterone can cause something called estrogen dominance. This is where a woman has far more estrogen but lower progesterone. Symptoms include hot flashes, night sweats, irritability, low libido, heavy periods, irregular periods, bloating, weight gain, hair loss, fatigue, brain fog, memory problems, fertility issues, and trouble sleeping.

Estrogen dominance can occur in one of two ways. First is inside the body when a woman's body makes too much estrogen and it cannot be metabolized. The second is caused by exposure to artificial estrogen (xenoestrogen) in the environment that cannot be properly detoxified from the body. In chapter 8, we will explore detoxification further, when we discuss the role of fiber intake. Factors that can contribute to an imbalance include:

- A sluggish impaired liver. The liver helps the body eliminate excess estrogen through the bowels. However, if liver detoxification is impaired by constipation, poor quality nutrition and imbalances in the gut microbiome, those estrogens can recirculate through the body.

- Stress causes the secretion of cortisol. This may cause the adrenal glands to suppress the production of progesterone in order to produce enough cortisol for the stressful event.
- Alcohol use, which can cause the circulating levels of estrogen in women to be higher. In addition, damage to the liver can negatively affect estrogen excretion.
- Excess caffeine, which can increase estrogen production.
- The estrobolome, a group of friendly bacteria in the microbiome that can metabolize and eliminate excess estrogen. They produce an enzyme that keeps estrogen in balance. However, conditions like dysbiosis of the gut cause the enzyme to get too high or out of balance. As a result, estrogen is not properly metabolized. This can lead to estrogen dominance.
- Xenoestrogens are foreign estrogens from our toxic environment that can block and bind receptors. They mimic our natural estrogen, causing imbalances and making a woman susceptible to estrogen dominance. They are found in plastics, milk and meat from cows fed hormones, self-care products, and pesticides. They become lodged in our fat cells and have been linked to diabetes, endometriosis, miscarriages, infertility, breast cancer, and obesity.

Testosterone

Testosterone is known as the libido hormone. However, because of societal norms, it's often associated with men. It's known as an androgen, which is a class of hormones found in higher amounts in men. However, women have these hormones as well.

As women, our testosterone levels are much lower than that of men. Yet, the amount we do have is vital for sexual desire, building bone, bone protection, energy, memory, motivation, confidence, and a sense of wellbeing.

Estradiol (E2) must be present in high enough levels for testosterone to perform at its optimum. If you don't have enough estrogen, testosterone cannot attach to your brain receptors.

Testosterone peaks at about age 25 and then gradually declines. At menopause testosterone declines by half, making it difficult to build muscle, resulting in increased body fat and problems with blood sugar control and metabolism. A decline in testosterone also lowers your sex drive.

If you are insulin resistant, you may have testosterone levels that are too high in relationship to other hormones such as estrogen. Addressing blood glucose levels can help to bring back the balance.

There are many ways to naturally increase testosterone, for example:

- Strength training
- HIIT (high intensity interval training)
- Vitamin D
- Quality sleep
- Stress management

- Intermittent fasting
  - Lowers levels of leptin, the hunger hormone, causing increased testosterone (according to *The Journal of Clinical Endocrinology and Metabolism*)
  - Can balance insulin, which, in turn, can improve testosterone levels

DHEA

DHEA is an androgen produced by the adrenal glands, the brain, and the spinal cord. It is the building block for 18 hormones, including estrogen and testosterone. It is the most abundant hormone in your body. DHEA promotes lean muscle, eases stress, improves your skin, helps you burn fat, improves memory, and supports bone growth. It peaks between the ages of 20 to 25. Thereafter, it declines by about 10 percent each year. Many women feel the effects of this decline in perimenopause when they experience vaginal and skin dryness, mood problems, weight gain, poor sleep, brain fog, and low libido.

Lower DHEA levels put you at risk for osteoporosis and heart disease. If you are under chronic stress with high cortisol levels, the production of DHEA is impacted. You become more vulnerable to insulin resistance. Low levels of DHEA cause higher insulin, and higher insulin will cause lower DHEA.

A healthy lifestyle can balance DHEA levels. A healthy diet that does not contain sugar and processed carbohydrates can improve your DHEA levels. The Okinawans in Japan have more DHEA in their bodies at age 65 and above than Americans of the same age because they are more likely to eat a natural diet and have times of fasting.

Thyroid Hormones

Your thyroid is on the front lower part of your neck. It is a metabolic regulator that is a key player in cellular function. It produces thyroxine (T4) and triiodothyronine (T3). T4 can convert to T3, which is the active form of the hormone.

Thyroid hormones help with the metabolism of protein, fat, and carbohydrates. They affect weight control, regulate energy levels, and support the mitochondria (an organelle found in most cells where the processes of energy production and respiration occur). Thyroid hormones also regulate internal temperature and help with tissue repair. An imbalance of the thyroid hormones affects every metabolic function in the body.

In perimenopause and menopause, thyroid problems can occur because of imbalances in estrogen and testosterone. This is because there are thyroid receptors on your ovaries, and your thyroid gland has ovary receptors, so the two work together.

Many women in perimenopause and menopause develop hypothyroidism, an underactive thyroid. Most of these cases are a result of Hashimoto's thyroiditis, an autoimmune disorder where the immune system attacks the thyroid and creates chronic inflammation. It is eight times more common in women than in men.

Both Hashimoto's and non-autoimmune hypothyroidism can be improved by treating nutrient deficiencies, infections, and food sensitivities. Identifying and treating toxins can also help in reversing symptoms.

Graves' disease is caused by an overactive thyroid (hyperthyroidism) and affects two to three percent of the population. It is an autoimmune disease resulting in abnormal enlargement of the thyroid gland (goiter). It can be treated with medication and diet.

With any thyroid disorder, a nutrient-dense whole-food diet combined with stress management and quality sleep is key. Balanced meals of protein, carbohydrates, and fats can improve thyroid function.

Intermittent fasting can potentially help by lowering insulin, which, in turn, can lower inflammation. However, in some individuals this could place too much hormetic stress on the body. If you are considering fasting and you have a thyroid disorder, work closely with your healthcare provider to determine if it's right for you. There are some people with thyroid issues who can successfully fast as long as nutrition, stress, and sleep are dialed in to optimum levels.

Growth Hormone

Growth hormone (GH) is produced by the pituitary gland and affects every cell in the body. It slows the aging process because it is important for cell growth, regeneration, and repair. GH builds greater bone density, builds and maintains muscle mass, gives you more energy, increases cognitive clarity, helps immunity, and improves the elasticity of your skin.

GH peaks in your early twenties and declines as you age. At age 50, you will have about half the amount you had in your twenties. This can cause muscle mass decrease, body fat increase, and bone loss.

Lifestyle habits that affect GH levels, either positively or negatively, include:

- GH is released overnight before waking in the morning. Thus, optimizing your sleep can boost levels.

- People with higher belly fat have lower levels of growth hormone.
- Higher insulin is linked to lower growth hormone levels. Eliminate sugar and late-night eating, which spikes insulin.
- HIIT (high intensity interval training) can boost GH.
- Intermittent fasting generally lowers insulin and increases GH according to a study where people fasted for two days.

Hormone Imbalance and Testing

When you're dealing with symptoms of hormone imbalance, such as weight gain, hot flashes, fatigue, and low libido, it's important to get your hormones tested, so you know what you need to change. Be sure to always discuss your hormone testing options with your healthcare provider.

There are three things to consider when testing your hormones. First, women's hormone testing is generally focusing only on sex, adrenal, and thyroid hormones. Second, normal ranges for test results vary and may not be your normal. If you have a number at the higher or lower end, you should discuss it with your trusted healthcare provider. Third, there is no one, single comprehensive test that will tell you everything you need to know.

Here are a few tests to consider with ranges suggested by the medical community:

- CBC Complete Blood Count

  o Red blood cells (RBC)—*4 million to 5 million cells/mcL.* Red blood cells carry oxygen and filter carbon dioxide, which means that a good number of them suggest your body is being well fueled. Too low a number can indicate anemia.

○ White blood cells (WBC) *4,500 to 10,000 cells/mcL*. White blood cells help your body to fight infection. High levels can indicate inflammation or infection in your body. Low levels show immune system problems.

○ Platelets—*140,000 to 450,000 cells/mcL*. Platelets help your blood to clot.

○ Hemoglobin (Hb or Hgb)—*12 to 15 gm/dL*. Hemoglobin is a protein that holds oxygen.

○ Hematocrit (Hct)—*36 percent to 44 percent*, which is the percentage of red blood cells to total blood. A low Hct score indicates you need iron while a high score can mean dehydration or other issues.

○ Mean corpuscular volume (MCV)—*80 to 95*. MCV refers to the average size of the red blood cells. Larger-than-normal cells can indicate a vitamin or folate deficiency while a smaller size indicates a form of anemia.

• Sex Hormones
Your hormone levels will fluctuate through each phase of your menstrual cycle. The levels listed are ranges within each phase and should indicate which phase you are currently in.

○ Estrone (E1) influences tissue growth and protects the heart, blood vessels, and brain. It can contribute to estrogen dominance. Levels fluctuate with the menstrual stage.

<200 pg/mL Luteal phase

<150 pg/mL Early follicular phase

25

100–250 pg/mL Follicular phase

3–32 pg/mL Post-menopausal

<150 pg/mL Non-pregnant

○ Estradiol (E2) is the strongest and purest estrogen in the body that helps with blood vessels, cholesterol, skin health, brain function, and immune system support. It must be properly balanced with progesterone and other estrogens to avoid estrogen dominance.

27–246 pg/mL Luteal phase

0–246 pg/mL Follicular phase

0–30 pg/mL Post-menopausal (untreated)

0–93 pg/mL Post-menopausal (treated)

0–102 pg/mL Oral contraceptive

○ Estriol (E3) is the unconjugated, normally weaker form of estrogen that increases during pregnancy and protects breasts, lungs, and digestion. It has anti-inflammatory qualities.

<0.08 ng/mL Non-pregnant

○ Progesterone balances estrogen throughout the body and supports the reproductive system. It affects bone, skin, mood, and brain health and is necessary for cortisol and thyroid balance.

0.72–17.8 ng/mL Luteal phase

0.33–1.2 ng/mL Follicular phase

0–1.0 ng/mL Post-menopausal

0.34–0.92 ng/mL Oral contraceptives

○ Testosterone is a powerful steroid hormone affecting libido, muscle mass, bone health, and hormonal balance. It can convert to estrogen. Measure both the total testosterone and the free testosterone to determine what is available in the body.

Total Testosterone

0–73 ng/dL Ovulating

0–43 ng/dL Post-menopausal

Free Testosterone

0.3–1.9 ng/dL

- Sex hormone-binding globulin (SHBG) is a protein produced in the liver that binds estrogen and testosterone within the bloodstream to keep the levels balanced.

  18–144 nmol/L Normal range

- Follicle-stimulating hormone (FSH) triggers estrogen production and is used to show ovarian function. Levels increase during ovulation and during ovarian failure. It can reveal signs of menopause.

  1.2–90 mlU/mL Luteal phase

  2.8–11.3 mlU/mL Follicular phase

  21.7–153.0 mlU/mL Post-menopausal untreated

  9.7–11.0 mlU/mL Post-menopausal treated

  0–4.9 mlU/mL Oral contraceptives

- Luteinizing hormone (LH) triggers ovulation and combines with FSH to promote fertility. It increases mid-cycle to stimulate the release of progesterone and to regulate ovarian estrogen production. It is influenced by prolactin levels. High levels are normal during menopause.

  0–14.7 mlU/mL Luteal phase

  1.1–11.6 mlU/mL Follicular phase

11.3–39.8 mlU/mL Post-menopausal

0–8.0 mlU/mL Oral contraceptives

- Cortisol levels show how your body is responding to stress. Because the levels fluctuate throughout the day, cortisol is best measured by blood in the morning and saliva four times throughout the day.

    Serum cortisol in the morning—this glucocorticoid hormone is released from the adrenal cortex and shows how well you handle stress.

    10–20 mcg/dL

    Four diurnal cortisol—tested four times per day with saliva.

    3.1–22.4 ng/dL

- DHEA is the most abundant sex hormone in the body, affecting cognition, the immune system, bone health, and aging. It is the precursor to estrogen and testosterone. Menstruation will affect its levels.

    35–430 ng/dL

- Insulin-like growth factor (IGF-1), produced by the liver, is the primary mediator of growth hormone (GH). It promotes cell growth, including skin, muscles, bones, and other organs.

    57–241 ng/mL

- Androstenedione is a steroid hormone that contributes to testosterone levels in the bloodstream and promotes muscle growth while supporting estrogen and testosterone levels.

    0.3–3.3 ng/mL

- Prolactin keeps other hormones in balance by inhibiting their production. It helps to regulate inflammation and metabolic processes as well as the metabolization of calcium. It stimulates breast milk production in lactating women.

  1.9–23.1 ng/mL

- Thyroid:

  ○ T3 is the active form of the thyroid hormone affecting heart rate, body temperature, and metabolism.

  100–180 ng/dL

  ○ Free T3 is the active form of the thyroid hormone, impacting metabolism. It is unbound and available in your bloodstream.

  2.5–4.4 pg/mL

  ○ Thyroid-stimulating hormone (TSH) shows how the brain is communicating with the thyroid.

  0.500–2.00 ulU/mL

  ○ Thyroxine (T4) is the main thyroid hormone in its inactive form for storage. It must be converted to T3 by the liver and the kidneys.

  6.0–12.0 ug/dL

  ○ Reverse T3 is an inactive form of the thyroid hormone. Increased levels can indicate inflammation and adrenal issues.

  9.0–21.0 ng/dL

  ○ Thyroid peroxidase antibody (TPOAb) is a thyroid antibody in the blood indicating the immune system is attacking the thyroid and that there could be an autoimmune disorder.

0–20 IU/mL

- ○ AntiTg antibody is normally not found in the bloodstream. If it rises before problems with other thyroid hormones, that indicates there could be an autoimmune thyroid problem.

    <90 lu/mL

- ○ Thyroxine (free T4) is the storage form of the thyroid hormone. After being triggered by TSH, T4 converts to T3, the active form of the thyroid hormone.

    1.00–1.50 ng/dL

- Fasting insulin/glucose—this test is used to diagnose prediabetes, diabetes, and metabolic syndrome. Insulin resistance affects cholesterol, blood glucose, and blood pressure.

    <90 mg/dL

- Hemoglobin A1C is hemoglobin with glucose attached to it. It helps evaluate your average glucose levels.

    4.8–5.6 percent

- HDL (cholesterol) is the "good cholesterol" that promotes heart health by aiding in the removal of harmful LDL cholesterol from the bloodstream by transporting it to the liver for excretion from the body.

    >39 mg/dL

- 25-Hydroxy vitamin D helps the body to absorb calcium for bone growth and other bodily functions.

    30.0–100.0 ng/mL

- Vitamin B12 promotes nerve and blood health as well as DNA production. It prevents anemia and keeps the blood balanced.

>150 ng/dL
- Folate is the natural form of vitamin B9 that is needed for cellular health and the synthesis of DNA and other genetic material.

2–20 ng/mL

Consult with your healthcare provider to determine what is best for you. Types of testing include:

- CBC (blood test)
- Thyroid (blood test)
- Adrenal (blood, saliva, and/or urine test)
- Sex hormones (blood, saliva, and/or urine test)
- Fasting insulin, glucose, HDL, hemoglobin A1C, IGF-1, 25-hydroxy-vitamin D, B12, and folate (blood test)

Clearly, hormonal imbalance can affect your ability to lose body fat and build muscle. However, through lifestyle habits such as nutrition, exercise, sleep, and stress management, you can reverse stubborn weight gain and restore your hormones to balance.

What I hope you are taking away from this chapter, and from the book overall, is that there is more to health and fitness for midlife women than the calories-in-and-calories-out model. In the next chapter, we look at how you can optimize your nutrition—not as a way to control calories—but as a means of balancing your hormones, which is key to the sound body and health you are seeking.

Chapter 3

Supporting Hormone Health with Nutrition

I met Shari for the first time on a Zoom consultation call. She was a beautiful, petite, 47-year-old woman with long blonde hair and green eyes. The first thing I noticed about Shari was that she appeared to be sad. She explained to me she was continually stressed trying to balance her job with raising two teen boys. She complained of poor sleep, low energy, and moodiness. However, her biggest concern was the excess body fat through her midsection.

After our call, Shari sent me current pictures, her weight, measurements, and health history. Although her weight appeared normal, I could tell from the photos and the waist and hip measurements that she had high body fat with low skeletal muscle mass. I created a plan for Shari, which focused on nutrition, resistance training, and improving her sleep.

Shari had been eating a low protein diet with high amounts of refined carbohydrates and very little healthy fat. She was also in the habit of snacking on sugary foods throughout the day and at night. We first focused on slowly increasing her protein intake. Protein is satiating and leaves less room for consuming the ultra-processed foods she was accustomed to eating.

Once Shari began to consistently hit her protein goal, I gradually helped her to swap out refined carbohydrates for natural whole food options, such as squash and low glycemic fruits. From there we decreased her intake of processed seed oils and replaced it with healthy fats, such as avocados, nuts, and seeds. Finally, we added in the balance component. This stage emphasized the best ratio of protein, carbs, and fats.

In six months, Shari changed the shape of her body. Her waistline decreased. The lower belly fat diminished. The shape of her glutes improved, her legs and shoulders were defined, and her body had symmetry. Her sleep, mood, and energy improved.

In my experience, most midlife women, like Shari, are not consuming nearly enough protein. As we move through this chapter, you will see that adequate quality protein combined with the right type and amount of carbohydrates and fats is the key to hormone balance and reducing body fat in the perimenopausal and menopausal years.

I remember getting up early to get my three children ready for school. The two youngest were picked up by the elementary school bus promptly at 7:15, and I drove my seventh-grade daughter to the local middle school. I would then come home and wash down a muffin with a cup of black coffee.

Then it was time for my morning run, which was anywhere from eight to 22 miles, depending on where I was in my marathon training. I would come back from those runs famished. The next meal was typically a grilled cheese sandwich or peanut butter on toast with a diet Coke. Somewhere in my 47 years, I had heard that cheese and peanut butter were great ways to get in my protein.

Fourteen years later, there is far more information available to us on nutrition. Social media platforms are littered with pictures of healthy recipes. However, I still find that women are confused about what to eat and how much (as I once was). This is especially true of women in midlife. The term "macronutrient" refers to a type of food—fat, protein, or carbohydrate—required in large amounts in the diet, and through my experience coaching, I've discovered that women are generally deficient in one main macronutrient—protein. When I first have clients track their food in an app, such as MyFitnessPal, most of the women are shocked to find their protein is low and nowhere near the number needed to build and maintain muscle.

All lifestyle changes start with proper nutrition, and your food choices are critical for reaching your fitness goals and for your health and wellness. Macronutrients—protein, carbohydrates, and fat—are all required in a nutritious eating plan. Micronutrients provide the vitamins and minerals your body needs whereas macronutrients provide the components for energy and maintaining the body's structure and systems. Understanding each macro is important for understanding the whole nutrition picture.

In this chapter, you'll learn the importance of tracking macronutrients (protein, fats, and carbohydrates). I will be providing you with specific food suggestions and a shopping list. We will also address the role of food sensitivities and glucose testing in improving our health in perimenopause and menopause.

Protein

Protein is the building block of muscle and the foundation for good health. The word "protein" comes from the Greek word πρώτειος (*proteios*), meaning "primary" or "first place."

Protein is found in animal products but is also present in other foods, such as nuts, cheese, and legumes. Protein is composed of 20 compounds called amino acids. Nine of these are considered essential because our body cannot make them. They must be obtained from food.

Protein does the following:

- Promotes growth and maintenance of body cells and tissues
- Builds and maintains muscle
- Is a building block for hormones
- Strengthens the immune system
- Makes you feel satiated and full after a meal
- Transports and stores nutrients
- Gives you energy
- Maintains the proper pH in the body (alkalinity and acidity)
- Stimulates biochemical reactions with enzymes, which are specialized proteins that regulate muscle contraction, blood clotting, digestion, and energy.

When working with midlife women, building muscle is my primary focus. Muscles are the largest site for the disposing of glucose (blood sugar), cholesterol, and fatty acid oxidation. As we age, we lose muscle (sarcopenia). Consuming adequate quality protein helps prevent and slow the loss of muscle tissue. The body needs amino acids to build and preserve muscle tissue and to prevent sarcopenia.

Sarcopenia begins around age 35 and occurs at a rate of one to two percent a year. It is the primary reason for age-related frailty and weakness in women. According to an article published in *PubMed*, when women lose the protection of estradiol in menopause, they can also lose skeletal muscle mass and strength. This is believed to be associated with a

Carol Covino

decline in estrogen, which could lead to an increase in visceral body fat and a decrease in bone density, muscle mass, and muscle strength.

Sarcopenia is accelerated by low levels of physical activity and low protein intake. Preventing sarcopenia is important for preventing functional impairment and physical disability.

Most American women do not eat enough protein to build and maintain muscle tissue and to sustain an ideal body weight. The standard American diet (SAD) is low in protein and high in processed grains, refined sugar, and seed oils. This does not support a healthy body composition.

My clients are surprised when I tell them how much protein they need to eat. There are a few different ways to calculate this. I find that one gram of protein per pound of ideal body weight is an adequate amount of protein to preserve muscle. If your healthy weight for your height and frame is 140 pounds, you need 140 grams of protein per day. Initially this number may seem overwhelming and impossible to meet. However, with a few dietary adjustments you can satisfy your body's protein needs.

Quality Protein

In general, you should eat a variety of grass-fed, organic, pasture-raised animal protein. My husband and I eat bison, grass-fed beef, buffalo, elk, and wild-caught fish and shellfish. I make it a habit to start my plate with quality protein, followed by healthy fat, vegetables, and finally a low-sugar-impact carbohydrate. I also eat my food in this same sequence to avoid blood sugar spikes. It's always protein first, followed by fat and vegetables, and my carbohydrate is eaten last. The past two months, I have been wearing a continuous glucose monitor (CGM) to see the impact of food and lifestyle habits on my glucose levels. I have found that eating in this order of protein first and carbs last has resulted in a lower blood sugar spike after meals.

When choosing protein, you want to stay away from conventionally produced chicken and beef. Conventionally raised corn-fed meat contains less vitamin E and beta carotene, and has very little anti-inflammatory omega-3 fats. Studies have indicated that the fatty acid profile is altered under conventional animal food production (according to the *British Journal of Nutrition*). Conventional chicken often contains antibiotic residue and unwanted pathogens, such as salmonella and E. coli. They can also contain chemical residue from pesticides.

Quality animal protein has the highest amino acid profile and is best for supporting the growth and repair of muscles and hormones. It's best to consume grass-fed beef, wild meats such as lamb, elk, buffalo, bison, and wild-caught fish from a reputable source such as Vital Choice Seafoods. If chicken is part of your diet, choose pasture-raised and antibiotic-free.

Saturated Fat in Meat

The saturated fat in red meat and other foods is often associated with elevated risk for heart disease, the leading cause of death for women in the United States. However, risk factors are being overweight or obese, smoking, not exercising, an unhealthy diet, and too much alcohol. The debate over saturated fat and heart disease is one of the most controversial topics in nutrition, and research has not been conclusive. A 2015 review looked at 15 randomized controlled trials with over 59,000 participants. It found that there were no significant effects of reducing saturated fat as it relates to preventing heart attacks, strokes, and death. In other words, those who reduced their intake of saturated fats were just as likely to die from heart attack or stroke as those who ate more saturated fat.

However, saturated fat tends to raise LDL (low-density lipoprotein) cholesterol, and high LDL is associated with an increased risk of heart disease and stroke. Many feel that the studies on saturated fat are not conclusive because they don't take into account the lifetime consumption of saturated fats. I personally choose to limit the amount of saturated fat in my diet to mitigate any risk.

The source of the saturated fats is believed to be very important in determining heart health. If the source of saturated fats is fast food, highly processed meats, fried food, and processed baked goods, it can affect health differently than a diet where saturated fats come from grass-fed meat or coconut. If you are at risk for high blood sugar (glucose), weight issues, and heart disease, talk to your doctor or cardiologist about this.

Vegan Protein

I understand that there may be religious, spiritual, or ethical reasons for not consuming animal protein. There are a variety of plant-based proteins available, including nuts, seeds, quinoa, beans, and legumes. However, it's important to understand that the quality of the protein from these sources is different from animal-based protein sources.

It is possible to obtain the essential amino acids from plants, but you need to consume a large amount of plant food to get the same amount of protein found in beef or other sources. For example, you would need to have five cups of quinoa to equal 40 grams of protein found in a five-ounce piece of lean beef. This would result in consuming 1,110 calories and 195 grams of carbohydrates.

One source of plant-based protein is soy found in tofu, edamame, vegan protein, and plant-based protein bars. Be aware that soy can mimic estrogen in the body and contribute to estrogen dominance. If you have a family history of cancer influenced by estrogen (for example, breast cancer), you may want to avoid soy. If you choose to have soy in your diet, consider organic fermented versions like miso and tempeh. Fermenting helps to neutralize the anti-nutrients.

There are additional problems with soy, including:

- Autoimmune thyroid disease because of the anti-nutrients, including phytates, which block the absorption of selenium
- Weight-loss resistance from inflammation due to a soy sensitivity. Many people are sensitive to soy.
- Headaches
- Fatigue
- Reproductive disorders
- Cognitive decline
- Digestive issues
- Lower sperm count

Soy is relatively new to America and 90 percent is genetically modified. Most soy produced in America is also heavily sprayed with pesticides. You may be thinking about Asia. People eat soy in Asia. In many of these countries, such as Japan, soy is more of a condiment and not the main ingredient or source of food. In America, soy is often converted to sausage, burgers, and other fake meats with added sugar, seed oils, and gluten.

Protein powder made from soy or hemp was found by the Clean Label Project to contain twice as much lead and higher amounts of contaminants than those made from animal sources. The article published in *Consumer Reports* noted that buying organic did not reduce the chances of contaminant exposure. Organic protein supplements actually had higher levels of heavy metals on average than nonorganic sources.

Fats

Our bodies need fat for fuel and for brain and heart health. They provide essential fatty acids that are protective to the body. Fats also do the following:
- Regulate leptin, so your brain knows you're full
- Give you energy
- Transport and distributes fat-soluble vitamins (A, D, E, K)
- Insulate and protect your body
- Form cellular membranes
- Are required for hormone production and regulation

Fats play a role in hormone balance and regulation. Most hormones are secreted by glands. However, some such as estrogen are produced in fatty tissue.

Cholesterol has a role with our sex hormones. The body can't produce progesterone, testosterone, and estrogen without it. The body produces cholesterol from dietary fat. Although high cholesterol has been associated with health fears, low cholesterol can cause health problems such as hormone imbalance and cognitive decline.

However, we should not consume just any fat source. We need to eat the "right" kinds of fats that contain omega-3 fatty acids. These include avocados, coconut oil, olive oil, nuts, nut butters, fatty fish, flaxseeds, and pasture-raised eggs (if you are not sensitive to eggs). There are unprocessed saturated fats, which are healthy choices. These include lean, grass-fed sources. Some saturated fats can help your body burn fat.

What about saturated fats and its association with heart disease? The source of saturated fats matters. A diet composed of fast foods, processed meats, and fried products will most likely have a different effect than eating saturated fats from grass-fed meat. Recent research surrounding saturated fats and heart disease has been controversial. However, we do know that being obese, eating an unhealthy diet, smoking, and lack of exercise increase the risk of death from heart disease in women.

Cholesterol travels through the blood on proteins called lipoproteins. There are two types of lipoproteins, low-density and high-density cholesterol. Low-density lipoproteins (LDL) make up most of the body's cholesterol, and high levels can raise the risk of heart disease and stroke. High-density lipoproteins (HDL) absorb cholesterol and carry it back to the liver where it is flushed from the body. HDL can lower your risk for heart disease.

Although eating saturated fat can increase LDL cholesterol, this often also results in higher HDL cholesterol and a decrease in triglycerides. The problem comes from the source of saturated fats. Highly processed foods, such as many of the packaged snacks found in the grocery stores, have been found to increase LDL cholesterol. I believe moderation is key. If you are at high risk, talk to your doctor or cardiologist about incorporating lean, grass-fed meats once or twice a week.

Saturated fat is also found in full-fat dairy products and eggs. Dairy products—including eggs—can be problematic for many midlife women who are struggling to lose weight, especially around the midsection. Although eggs contain key nutrients, many people are sensitive to them. They can cause bloating, gas, diarrhea, abdominal pain, and other digestive issues. Dairy produced in the United States contains several hormones that are detrimental to our health. It also contains lactose, which can cause digestive problems, gas, and bloating. Here are just a few reasons midlife women should consider eliminating dairy:

- It can raise insulin levels, which is associated with insulin resistance and weight gain.
- It causes belly bloating due to lactose.
- It can contain synthetic versions of bovine growth hormone (rBGH).
- It exposes us to antibiotics given to cows.
- It raises IGF-1, which has been associated with an elevated risk of cancer.
- It has components which mimic morphine, making it addictive. A milk protein called casein is broken down into casomorphins, which are morphine-like proteins that cross the blood-brain barrier and contribute to the release of dopamine. Dopamine is the pleasure center of the brain. For this reason, many researchers refer to dairy products as "dairy crack."

Polyunsaturated fats found in vegetable and seed oils should be avoided. They are high in omega-6 fatty acids, which are inflammatory and increase free radicals in the body. Free radicals are molecules that contain oxygen and have an uneven number of electrons. The uneven number allows them to react with other molecules. They can cause large chain chemical reactions in your body because of these reactions with other molecules. These reactions are called oxidation and can damage cells, causing illness, disease, and aging.

According to Dr. Catherine Shanahan, seed oils can affect the health of your cellular membranes and mitochondria, causing damage which lasts up to two years. The mitochondria are responsible for many functions, including respiration and energy production. They basically power the cell's biochemical reactions and make most of the cell's supply of adenosine triphosphate (ATP), a molecule used for energy. We will be discussing mitochondria throughout this book. They are critical for understanding metabolic and cellular health.

Avoid these seven oils:

- Canola
- Corn
- Cottonseed
- Peanut
- Safflower
- Soybean
- Sunflower

Vegetable oils can also increase hunger and cravings. Vegetable oil can trigger something called endocannabinoid overactivity when hunger-promoting receptors in the hypothalamus are activated. The linoleic acid is a precursor for molecules that activate the hunger centers of the brain. Our body fat has 10 to 20 times the linoleic acid concentration of body fat from over a hundred years ago (a time prior to vegetable oils). As mentioned above, linoleic acid also shuts down energy production. Thus, there is the potential for low energy combined with high hunger.

It bears mentioning that there are discrepancies between doctors, researchers, and nutritionists concerning the consumption of these oils. Some say that canola oil can be a healthy addition to the diet. However, I believe that the circumstances under which these oils are produced make them a poor fat choice. Watch a video on how canola oil is made to see what I mean.

In addition, researchers have connected soybean oil with cognitive disorders, such as autism, Alzheimer's disease, anxiety, and depression. It also has been linked to obesity and diabetes. These oils are found just about everywhere and are commonly used in restaurants because they are less expensive options. Even upper-end steakhouses often use seed oils to cook the meat.

Healthy Fat Choices

Healthy fats are found in nuts, seeds, organic cold-pressed extra-virgin olive oil, avocados, organic cold-pressed coconut oil, and fatty fish such as wild Alaskan salmon. Olive oil and avocado have monounsaturated fat, which can reduce inflammation and guard against inflammation. Some coconut oils have medium-chain triglycerides that stimulate your liver to burn stored fat for energy (in particular, stored abdominal fat).

Including 12 ounces of omega-3 rich seafood in your weekly eating plan can help reduce the joint pain associated with inflammation and autoimmune disease. It's important to distinguish between omega-6 and omega-3 fats. Omega-6 fats are associated with inflammation. The ratio of omega-3 to omega-6 fats in the diet should be one-to-one. Most Americans eat far too many omega-6 fats and not enough omega-3 fats in their diet. The standard American diet ratio is 20-to-one (omega-6 to omega-3).

Carbohydrates

Carbohydrates produce the most confusion. Should you eat carbs? How many carbs should you consume? Is low carb better? What about no carb?

There are the following three main types of carbohydrates:

- Sugars—these include glucose, fructose, sucrose, and galactose. They are constructed of single or double molecules.
- Starches—these are multiple sugar molecules that get broken down into glucose during digestion.
- Fiber—this is the non-digestible part of plants that can feed the healthy bacteria in the gut, lower glucose and fat absorption, and aid in weight control.

There are whole and refined carbohydrates. Whole carbs are unprocessed and have not been refined. Refined carbohydrates are processed and have had the natural fiber removed or altered.

Whole carbohydrates include quinoa, legumes, potatoes, sweet potatoes, whole grains, and winter squash. They are high in fiber, rich in nutrients, and can aid in removing harmful estrogen from the body.

Refined carbohydrates are high in sugar and include white flour products, white bread, jams, candy, syrup, table sugar, and many processed foods. They are high in calories and low in nutrients. They can increase inflammation, cause food cravings, elevate blood glucose (sugar), contribute to metabolic inflexibility, and negatively impact the gut microbiome.

About Low Carb

I have found from working with over a thousand women that the amount of carbohydrates needed depends on the individual. For this reason, I do not make specific recommendations without knowing someone's bio-individual needs. However, there are times when a lower carbohydrate nutrition plan can be beneficial.

If you are insulin resistant, a low-carb diet combined with intermittent fasting can help reduce insulin levels and stabilize blood sugar.

If you have a large amount of weight to lose, a lower carb eating plan will help your body to burn its fat reserves for energy rather than its stored carbohydrates. Carbohydrates are a quick form of energy. If you have a large amount stored, your body will burn the carbs instead of the stored fat. This creates metabolic flexibility.

Leptin resistance occurs when you overeat and leptin levels are continually high. Over time, your brain does not recognize the signal from your body that it's full. This is called leptin resistance. It can be reversed with a lower carbohydrate diet. When you lose weight, your leptin levels drop, and your cells are no longer resistant to leptin.

There are women who cannot tolerate a low-carb diet for long periods of time because it can potentially have a negative impact on thyroid function. This is why it's important to do some self-testing in terms of how many carbohydrates you can eat daily, a subject you'll read about shortly. Also, low-carbohydrate plans can be restrictive and difficult to sustain for more than a few weeks at a time.

About Carb Cycling

I have found that cycling on and off carbs, "carb cycling," can be beneficial. With carb cycling you alternate higher carbohydrate intake with lower carbohydrate intake. This can be done on a weekly or monthly rotation.

- Carb cycling is easier to maintain as opposed to a strictly low-carb or ketogenic diet, because it provides more flexibility and a greater selection of foods. On a low-carb diet you are limited to certain vegetables and little to no fruit.

- Carb cycling replenishes muscle glycogen, which is diminished by low-carb diets and exercise.
- It can increase metabolism by assisting with the conversion of the inactive thyroid hormone T4 to the active form of T3.
- It promotes metabolic flexibility, allowing your body to be efficient at both burning fat and carbohydrates for fuel.
- It sends a message to the body that it's not starving, which can increase fat burning and help to break weight loss plateaus.
- It regulates the hunger hormones ghrelin and leptin, which helps you control your appetite.
- It can improve insulin sensitivity by balancing insulin.

How many carbohydrates you consume on your lower and higher carb days is bio-individual and varies based on activity level, age, fitness goals, and even genetics. On lower carbohydrate days, you will have your carb intake at about 25 percent of your daily calories. Typically, this is going to be under 90 grams per day. On higher carbohydrate days, you will increase your intake to be about 50 percent of your daily caloric intake, which will generally be 140 to 180 grams per day. Again, this is highly dependent on the individual and their activity level. My low carb day may be much higher or lower than your low carb day.

Self-Testing Your Glucose Levels

As I write this book, I am wearing a continuous glucose monitor (CGM) to check my glucose (blood sugar) levels and how my body responds to different foods, intermittent fasting periods, and to exercise. I am using the Nutrisense CGM, which is simple to use and pain free to apply. According to functional medicine practitioners, your fasted morning blood sugar level should be in the range of 80–95 mg/DL or less. The fasting level is determined by at least an eight-hour overnight period where you are not consuming food or drinks. Glucose floats on top of all the fat in your body. Measuring your blood sugar when you wake up or before you eat a meal is a good way to be sure you are not continually consuming too many carbohydrates or fats.

Your goal is to have stability in your blood glucose. Consistent spikes of more than 30 points after a meal may be a sign that you have had too many carbohydrates. Reducing the amount of carbohydrates and increasing fat can be helpful. If your glucose continually spikes over 100, it could be caused by poor sleep, illness, or too many carbohydrates. If your number spikes 140 or more after a meal, it may be a sign of insulin resistance.

I have also been using my CGM to monitor my hunger cues. You can do this by checking your blood sugar levels when you feel hungry and then track your feelings over the course of three days. Record all the readings and obtain an average. The average is referred to as your "trigger point." Once you have completed the three-day test, check your glucose to see if you are at your trigger point. This means you need fuel (energy). If you are not at the trigger point, this means you still have energy to burn as fuel. You will wait to eat your next meal.

Your premeal blood glucose will generally be close to your waking blood glucose. This means that managing your blood sugar level before you eat is more useful for health and fat loss than being concerned with the spike after a meal. Check the levels after you eat. If your glucose rises less than 30 points, it means your protein, fat, and carbs are good. If it rises more than 30 points, you have had too many carbs and will need to adjust on the next meal.

About Carb Quality

When it comes to eating carbohydrates, know that whole unprocessed carbohydrates such as fruits and vegetables have anti-inflammatory properties and contain a variety of vitamins and minerals that can protect against cellular damage. Green vegetables contain isoflavones, which help your liver excrete harmful, excess estrogen. Berries contain vitamin C, which helps your body fight inflammation. Therefore, all of these are high quality carbs.

There are some grains, which are considered to be healthy, including gluten-free oats, brown rice, wild rice, quinoa, and millet. However, if you have an autoimmune disease, it can be beneficial to eat a grain-free diet. In addition, you may not process grains as well past age 40. Since I have an autoimmune disease, rheumatoid arthritis, I opt to limit or avoid most grains. Most of my carbohydrates come from cooked starchy vegetables and fruits. Cooked starchy vegetables include:

- Beans
- Beets
- Carrots
- Green peas
- Lentils

- Parsnips
- Plantains—a starchy, tropical fruit related to the banana. They are usually cooked in the same way as potatoes.
- Pumpkin
- Sweet potato
- Winter squash—acorn or butternut squash

Resistant starch resists digestion in the small intestine and can result in better blood sugar and insulin control. Enzymes in the gastrointestinal (GI) tract are inactive against it. Once the resistant starch reaches the large intestine, it is fermented into short-chain fatty acids, which are used as fuel for beneficial microbes and enterocytes of the GI tract. We will be discussing fatty acids more in depth in chapter 8. This can support microbial balance and intestinal health. Examples of resistant starches include green plantains, beans, legumes, raw potato starch, and cooked and cooled sweet potatoes.

Carbohydrates are not "the devil." Rather, they can be a part of a sustainable nutrition plan when you are learning to choose the right kinds of carbs in the right amount for your body.

If you stick to the following three principles, you can incorporate carbohydrates without weight gain or blood glucose dysregulation:

- Slow-digesting carbs are the best option. As mentioned above, vegetables such as broccoli, beets, and carrots are a great carb to include in your meals. Beans and lentils are slow digesting as well. However, you will want to soak and pressure cook them to remove inflammatory lectins, especially if you have an autoimmune disease.

- The time of day you eat carbs is important to consider. The first meal of the day is the most important to be aware of. Eating too many carbohydrates, especially in the morning, can start the day on a "sugar rollercoaster ride." Putting off your carb intake until later in the day and then consuming the slow digesting carbs will help to regulate blood glucose levels.
- Match your carbohydrate intake to your age, stage of life, activity level, and health status. A 50-year-old insulin-resistant woman cannot eat as many carbs as a highly physically active woman in her thirties. Always consider bio-individuality. What works for one woman may not be the best option for another.

Your Macro Count

What should be your macro count, meaning the amount of protein, carbohydrates, and fat you should eat daily? There is no definitive answer to this question. Once again, it is dependent on the individual and their goals. There are many factors at play, including stage of life, hormones, activity level, and genetics. I generally set women a starting point of 40 percent protein, 25 percent carbs, and 35 percent fats, and adjust as needed.

It's important to keep track of how you feel on different macronutrient plans. You can do that by asking yourself the following questions and recording your responses:

- Are you continually tired?
- Do you feel more or less energetic after a meal?
- How is your sleep, mood, and mental clarity?

- What about your appetite? Are you satiated after each meal, or are you still hungry?
- Do you have sweet and salty cravings between meals?

Lisa came to me at age 55. She had been fit, athletic, and positive her entire life. She didn't believe menopause would change her body and mental outlook. Yet, after turning 50, she noticed a gradual shift in her body. She gained 20 pounds with much of the body fat settling in her mid-section. Her sleep began to suffer. She had hot flashes and felt irritable and depressed.

The loss of key hormones such as estrogen, progesterone, and testosterone along with her nutrition habits were the root cause. She wasn't eating the right proportion of protein, carbohydrates, and fats to support the hormonal shift that had occurred as she transitioned into menopause.

Her protein was too low. Her carbohydrate choices were poor and her carb consumption too high. She wasn't consuming enough healthy fats. I reduced her carbs and increased her protein and fat intake so that her macro count was 45 percent protein, 30 percent fat, and 25 percent carbs. The macronutrient changes along with strength training resulted in Lisa losing 10 pounds, reducing her waistline, and feeling like her old energetic self again.

Your Grocery List

"What should be on my grocery list?" I am often asked this question. To repeat, as women we are bio-individually unique. However, there are a few general principles when it comes to food selection. Here goes:

Refrigerator
- Almond milk
- Asparagus
- Broccoli
- Brussel sprouts
- Carrots
- Cauliflower
- Celery
- Chives
- Coconut milk
- Dandelion greens
- Dijon mustard
- Garlic
- Green frozen bananas
- Guacamole
- Hummus
- Jicama tortillas
- Lemons
- Limes
- Mushrooms
- Nut butter
- Parsley
- Radishes
- Red onions
- Salad greens

Freezer
- Frozen wild-caught seafood, such as scallops, shrimp, salmon, cod, sole, halibut, and Alaskan crab
- Pasture-fed pork tenderloin
- Grass-fed beef and bison
- Organic free-range chicken and turkey
- Lamb

- Frozen wild berries, such as blueberries, strawberries, and raspberries
- Frozen vegetables

Pantry
- Almond flour
- Artichoke hearts (I love the ones from Trader Joes.)
- Balsamic vinegar (for salad dressing)
- Bone broth
- Cassava flour
- Coconut flour
- Coconut milk (full fat)
- Garbanzo beans
- Green tea
- Lentils
- Nuts (chestnuts, macadamia, pecans, pine nuts, pistachios, and walnuts)
- Quinoa
- Red curry coconut sauce (I recommend the kind made by Thai Kitchen.)

Vegetable Bin
- Avocados
- Beets
- Butternut squash
- Garlic
- Onions
- Shallots
- Sweet potatoes
- Turnips

Spices
- Basil
- Black pepper

- Cinnamon
- Cumin
- Curcumin
- Italian herbs
- Mexican spices
- Red chili
- Red pepper
- Rosemary
- Sea salt

Oils and Other Healthy Fats
- Avocado oil
- Chia seeds
- Coconut milk or cold-pressed organic oil
- Extra-virgin olive oil (I like the Olive Oil Club.)
- Flaxseed
- Grass-fed ghee and butter
- Hemp seeds
- MCT oil
- Olives
- Sesame oil
- Tahini

Food Sensitivity

Although many of the foods described in this chapter are nutritious, if you have leaky gut (intestinal permeability) or problems with food sensitivity, you could experience inflammation from even the healthiest of foods. Inflammation can also cause weight loss resistance and leptin resistance.

In chapter 2, we discussed the hormone leptin. Leptin is a hormone that responds to how much you've eaten and sends the satiety signal that you've had enough to eat. It also adjusts your metabolism to either slow down or to burn fat in order to keep your body in homeostasis. Leptin resistance makes it even more difficult to lose weight because you are not receiving the proper signals. Healing inflammation helps to remedy leptin resistance.

For this reason, it's important to consider keeping a food journal, doing an elimination diet, or having a lab sensitivity test to determine your food intolerance. If doing an elimination diet, you will want to take out eggs, corn, dairy, gluten, peanuts, sugar/artificial sweeteners, and soy. Eliminate these foods for 21 days. From there, you can gradually reintroduce one food at a time to see how your body responds. I recommend following the guidelines given in J.J. Virgin's book *The Virgin Diet*. You'll find comprehensive instructions on how to do this successfully.

Because I had to take immunosuppressant medications to control the symptoms of autoimmune disease, I have experienced problems in the past with gut dysbiosis, a condition where the gut bacteria become imbalanced. As a result, I developed several food intolerances. I learned that lectin is a common culprit for inflammation, and it is found in barley, beans, brown rice, dairy products, eggplant, cucumbers, lentils, peas, peanuts, potatoes, soy products, wheat, whole grains, and tomatoes. Soaking, peeling, deseeding, and pressure cooking in an InstaPot can significantly reduce or remove lectins.

There can also be genetic differences in how we process many healthy foods, including sulfur- and oxalate-containing vegetables. You could have a compromised sulfur metabolism, which results in bloating, gas, and malabsorption of nutrients. In addition, some individuals have a genetic predisposition to difficulty with metabolizing fat. Proper fat metabolism and absorption is critical to brain and cognitive function.

It's important to remember that we are bio-individually different. Having worked with over a thousand women over the past decade, I have found that I cannot make assumptions. Each woman has a unique set of circumstances, including health history, stage of life, hormones, and genetics. This is why having tests performed and read by a functional medicine practitioner may be beneficial. Tests such as the DUTCH (dried urine and saliva testing for hormones), the GI-MAP (DNA-based stool testing), and blood tests for food sensitivity can give greater insight into our overall health.

In the next chapter, we will be exploring the benefits of intermittent fasting and meal timing for midlife women. Intermittent fasting is not a diet with a set of fixed rules and dos and don'ts. Rather, it's part of a healthy lifestyle that provides flexibility with meal timing. The beauty of intermittent fasting is that you choose the fasting and feeding windows that work with your activity level, energy, sleep, and personal schedule.

Chapter 4

Age in Reverse With Intermittent Fasting

Ashley came to me wanting to lose 10 pounds. At 58, she was running close to 10 miles per day in an attempt to control her weight. She lacked muscle tone and carried a great deal of body fat in the lower belly. She first joined one of my challenges where the focus was on strength training. After six weeks, Ashley was excited to see muscle emerging in her arms and legs.

She then joined my six-week intermittent fasting program. This was where the magic occurred. On most days, Ashley ate dinner at 6:00 p.m. and broke her fast at 10:00 a.m. In her eight-hour feeding window, she consumed approximately 125 grams of protein, 65 grams of fat, and 105 grams of carbohydrates. Ashley's final meal typically consisted of five ounces of cooked lean protein such as a chicken breast, two cups of cruciferous vegetables such as cauliflower, and a half-cup of sweet potato or quinoa. A small amount of slow-acting carbohydrate helped Ashley with sleep and cortisol levels in the evening. Slow carbohydrates take more time to digest and do not cause the same rapid rise in blood sugar that refined carbs can cause. The right type of carbs can help stress levels by blunting the cortisol response. This allows the body to move into the parasympathetic mode for a more restful sleep. Ashley lost 10 pounds and reduced her waistline by three inches. More importantly, she shared with me how she had gained confidence, increased her energy level, and, in her words, became "happier."

The first time intermittent fasting came to my attention was about five years ago when I was sitting in a sauna at my gym. I remember the sauna was hotter than usual on that particular day. The sweat was pouring into my eyes, and I was counting the seconds until I could step out into the cooler air.

At that moment, a man sat down beside me, completely covered in long sweats and a thick hoodie pulled over his face. He was an MMA fighter. He struck up a conversation and began explaining how he had changed his diet to train for his next fight. He was using something called intermittent fasting. I was horrified as he described not eating for 18 hours and then breaking his fast with pizza and ice cream. As a fitness and nutrition coach this sounded like insanity to me.

It wasn't long after the sauna talk that a midlife woman contacted me for coaching. She wanted me to write an intermittent fasting plan for her. I told her that I did not believe in fasting and was unable to advocate that type of program.

A lot has changed in five years. What seemed like a new, radical fad diet to me is actually a practice, which has been done by human beings throughout time and has its roots firmly based in science. As mentioned in chapter 2, intermittent fasting is simply time-restricted eating. You fast or abstain from eating for a period of time. This is followed by a feeding window where you consume food. Intermittent fasting is done several different ways. It can include 12 hours of fasting followed by 12 hours where you consume your meals. The most common intermittent fasting schedule suggested for women over the age of 40 is 16:8. This is 16 hours where food is not eaten followed by an eight-hour period where meals are consumed.

Intermittent fasting is often distinguished from fasting. Many see fasting as a practice where you abstain from food for extended periods of time of 24 hours or more. In contrast, they define intermittent fasting as specific feeding and fasting windows within a 24-hour period or within a weekly schedule. Others do not make the distinction and use the terms intermittent fasting and fasting interchangeably. In this chapter, we are specifically referring to time-restricted eating or intermittent fasting. As you read further, you will gain a better understanding of this practice.

When intermittent fasting is properly done, it is not only safe but beneficial for many midlife women. It can burn stored fat, regenerate our cells, and stabilize our hormones, which decreases our likelihood of developing chronic diseases, such as autoimmune disorders, diabetes, and vascular disease.

The practice of intermittent fasting is similar to our ancestral eating patterns. Our ancient relatives did not eat three meals per day plus snacks. They did not have easy and unlimited access to food. They most likely didn't eat for long periods of time because food was not easily available. Eating varied according to the season. At times our ancestors may have eaten several times throughout the day, and at other times they would have only one meal or no food at all. Thus, intermittent fasting is not a new and novel phenomenon. It has been practiced by human beings throughout time; thus, we are born into bodies primed and ready to eat in this manner.

Intermittent fasting is a powerful tool we can use to prevent "metabolic inflexibility." According to the National Center for Health Statistics, obesity increased in women over 20 years old from 25.5 percent to 40.7 percent over the past few decades. In women 40 to 59 years of age, 61 percent are overweight or obese. Obesity is linked to devastating illnesses, such as type 2 diabetes, heart disease, and cancer, and it is one consequence of being metabolically inflexible. In 2017, only 12 percent of Americans were considered to be metabolically healthy. That number is estimated to be much lower in 2022. Metabolic inflexibility can lead to diseases, such as high blood pressure, inflammation, and insulin resistance.

Let's look at metabolic flexibility and inflexibility more, so you can better understand how intermittent fasting aids you. You want to be able to burn both fat and carbohydrates for energy. If you are not metabolically flexible, you will only burn sugar (carbs) for fuel and have a difficult time tapping into stored fat for energy. Your glucose levels will be more likely to rise higher than normal and remain high throughout the day. Over time, this can lead to poor metabolic markers such as high insulin and fasting glucose levels. Chronic diseases such as type 2 diabetes, cardiovascular, and fatty liver are linked with insulin resistance. Women approaching menopause are more likely to have a problem with glucose and insulin regulation, making them more vulnerable to chronic diseases, including those associated with cognitive decline. Thus, it's important to be metabolically flexible. Intermittent fasting is one powerful tool for fat burning and ensuring metabolic flexibility.

Intermittent fasting can balance hormones, create metabolic flexibility, give more mental clarity and focus, and increase energy. It can also help you to be more productive throughout the day because your schedule is no longer filled with planning meals and snacks. Being a bikini bodybuilder for the past decade, I was accustomed to eating six to seven small meals per day. I did not realize how much of my mental energy and time was wrapped up in planning and consuming these mini-meals until I began practicing intermittent fasting.

Intermittent fasting is based on time-restricted eating and meal timing. There is no one strategy to intermittent fasting. Rather, it should involve an individualized approach. An intermittent fasting plan should be different for women than men as our physiology is not like men's. We must take into account our life stage—child bearing, perimenopausal, menopausal, or beyond. Our hormones will fluctuate based on our life stage.

In this chapter you will learn the most common myths related to intermittent fasting, its definition, and how it can improve hormonal balance and health in women over the age of 40.

Myths Related to Fasting

Before we look at the different approaches to intermittent fasting and which one may be right for you, we need to unpack some of the myths and dogma surrounding women's health and weight loss that may be harmful.

Myth 1: Breakfast is the most important meal of the day.

We have been told that eating breakfast is a healthy thing to do and that skipping breakfast could lead to weight gain and health problems. My training in health and nutrition focused primarily on encouraging clients to eat breakfast within 20 to 40 minutes of rising and to never go past two to three hours before consuming the next meal. In fact, this is a mantra of the bodybuilding world.

The truth is that there is no real evidence to support this. A review of 13 clinical trials published between 1990 and 2018 found that breakfast might not be a good strategy for weight loss and that recommending breakfast for weight loss in adults could have the opposite result. The study also found that those who skipped breakfast weighed less than those who regularly ate breakfast.

Myth 2: Eating small meals throughout the day revs up your metabolism.

As mentioned already, this is a strong belief in the bodybuilding community. I started my fitness transformation by committing to compete in a bodybuilding show. The first thing my coach did was to write a meal plan, which consisted of six small meals throughout the day. Yes, I became lean. However, this had more to do with the amount of protein and the quality of foods I was eating. Gone was sugar and ultra-processed food. Protein became a priority.

For many years, I subscribed to the belief that eating multiple meals increases metabolism, burns more calories, and controls hunger. The reality is none of this is true. Studies have indicated that there is no weight loss benefit to splitting calories among six meals rather than three and that increasing meals from three to six does not stimulate fat loss. There is also no evidence that eating more frequently controls hunger. However, eating larger, less frequent meals can reduce hunger and increase satiety.

Another study found that people who were told to delay breakfast for 90 minutes and eat dinner 90 minutes earlier lost twice as much body fat as those who ate on their normal schedules. This fat loss occurred despite the subjects being allowed to eat what they wanted during their feeding window.

Myth 3: Calories are the most important thing for weight loss.

It's the quality of the food and the right proportion of macros (protein, carbohydrates, and fats) that is the primary focus for fat loss and weight control. Poor quality foods such as ultra-processed carbs and sweets are the main contributors to weight gain and metabolic inflexibility. However, it's not just the number of calories in these foods that causes weight gain. Rather, it's the physiological responses in the body, which cause fat storage. Ultra-processed carbs and sweets quickly break down into sugar. When this occurs, your pancreas creates higher levels of the hormone insulin. Insulin tells your body to convert calories to fat.

Studies have shown that when you consume whole foods in their natural state, it reduces the risk of chronic disease and improves health. Whole foods tend to be lower in sugar and higher in fiber. This helps to stabilize blood glucose levels and lower the fat-storing hormone insulin. Fiber slows down the glucose spikes, which occur after a meal. In addition, many whole foods such as vegetables and fruits often contain prebiotics and postbiotics, which improve the balance of the gut microbiome. When our gut has the right proportion of bacteria, fungi, and microbes, our immunity and digestion are improved. Whole foods are also nutrient dense providing the vitamins and minerals we need for overall health. They often contain the perfect combination of nutrients to facilitate absorption.

On the other hand, if we eat an ultra-processed diet, we are upsetting the delicate balance of the gut microbiome. Yeast overgrowth is a common problem leading to gut dysbiosis. The greater the overgrowth of yeast, the more we crave the very foods (sugar and refined carbs) that feed even more growth of yeast. Ultra-refined foods are also low in nutrients and high in calories.

Slashing calories sets off a reaction in the body, which slows metabolism and increases hunger. Our bodies are smart. When we drastically cut calories, our metabolism slows down to preserve food and energy longer. The hunger hormones ghrelin and leptin become imbalanced causing increased hunger.

Intermittent Fasting—What It Is

Intermittent fasting simply means that you are eating less often and within a time-restricted feeding window. During your feeding window, you should be choosing quality protein, healthy fats, and non-starchy carbs rather than focusing on a caloric amount.

There are different forms of intermittent fasting. One form of intermittent fasting is an alternate day schedule where you eat one day and fast the next. Another option is a five-to-two fasting plan where you fast two days per week and eat the other five days. The third is daily intermittent fasting where you go 12 to 16 hours or more without food and eat within a feeding window.

I have found with myself and in working with women that the daily intermittent fasting approach works best and is the simplest to implement. I encourage my clients to follow anywhere from the 12-to-12 model (12 hours fasting and 12 fed) to the 16-to-8 plan (16 hours fasting and eight fed). The time of day that you implement your fasting window depends on your schedule. For most women, the fasting window will begin in the evening. I suggest starting your fast by 7:00 pm after your last meal of the day. If you are following the 16-to-8 plan, you will break your fast at 11:00 a.m. (16 hours after 7:00 p.m.). Your feeding window would be from 11:00

a.m. to 7:00p.m. (eight hours). However, I have worked with night shift employees such as nurses who need to follow a different schedule. This is the beauty of intermittent fasting. It's flexible. You choose the fasting window that works with your lifestyle.

Specifically, the 16-to-8 model is generally the most flexible and beneficial plan for women of all ages. However, once again, this is bio-individual. I have clients who fast for 13, and 14 hours. I have others who do the 16-to-8 model during the week and do not fast on the weekends. Start small at 12 hours fasting, and gradually increase to 16.

Benefits of Intermittent Fasting

Intermittent fasting allows for many benefits. First and foremost, it creates metabolic flexibility. To review, metabolic flexibility is the ability of your cells to switch between using carbohydrates and fat for fuel. This means you can burn fat when you're not eating at all, or your body can burn both carbs and fat when eating. Your body is flexible and able to use whatever fuel is available from food or what is stored in your body.

When you are metabolically inflexible, you will have difficulty waiting to eat between meals. You may experience a shaky, nauseous feeling if you don't eat or snack frequently. It will be difficult, if not impossible, to lose weight and body fat because of the dysregulated glucose levels. The higher the blood sugar spikes, the more insulin that is required to clean up the mess. Insulin is a fat storing hormone. If you are releasing insulin, you are not burning fat. Chronically high insulin levels can lead to the body ceasing to recognize and respond to insulin. This leads to insulin resistance, prediabetes, and type 2 diabetes. Research studies are also beginning to link insulin resistance with Alzheimer's, dementia, and cognitive decline. Intermittent fasting improves metabolic flexibility by forcing the body to use fat stores for energy. Having times where you decrease carbohydrate intake can increase your ability to tap into fat stores, similar to how our ancestors needed to be efficient at burning fat during times of scarcity.

Our modern times have given people an abundance of processed food, and it is no longer necessary for our bodies to burn fat for fuel. This is a recipe for disaster. Our modern world collides with ancient physiological responses still present in our bodies. The production of insulin is believed to be a survival mechanism, which kept human beings alive in anticipation of long winters and food scarcity. From a survival perspective, it was to our benefit to have high insulin and store fat. In fact, we have a natural taste and desire for sweet foods because of this survival mechanism. Our ancestors would have consumed an abundance of fruits such as wild berries raising blood glucose levels, which would help them in times of scarcity. Today, winter is not coming, and for most Americans, the berries have been replaced with refined, sugary foods.

When we consume these foods, it ignites the survival pathway through the release of insulin. In response, our bodies store fat. Because there is an abundance of highly processed foods, which spike blood glucose, the body does not need to rely on fat for fuel. It has plenty of calories in the form of refined carbohydrates and high fructose corn syrup. According to Dr. David Perlmutter, a board-certified neurologist and author, the consumption of fructose corn syrup ignites a survival pathway through the production of uric acid. High uric acid has been associated with chronic metabolic degenerative diseases. The World Health Organization tells us this is the number one cause of death on our planet.

When you are metabolically flexible you will have balanced hormones, less sugar spikes, increased energy, fewer cravings, and a greater ability to burn fat. When exercising, you will generally be able to use fat as energy over carbs and have better performance and energy. When someone who is metabolically inflexible exercises, they cannot switch as easily to burning fat. They will burn more stored carbohydrates (glycogen) and reach fatigue quicker.

Another benefit with intermittent fasting is that it improves gut health. We have trillions of microorganisms living in our intestines. This is called the microbiome. These microorganisms break down food and nutrients and feed on fiber and forms of starch found in our foods. This allows the microbiome to create compounds that help prevent disease. The microbiome can also impact our mood by sending signals to the brain.

It's important for health to feed your gut bacteria what it needs to maintain the balance of good to bad microorganisms. The balance is also affected by meal timing. Fasting promotes an increase in the good microorganisms.

Intermittent fasting also supports the migrating motor complex (MMC). The MMC moves food and particles through the digestive tract. It helps to prevent gut infections and small intestinal bacterial overgrowth (SIBO). The MMC controls stomach and small intestine contractions over a period of approximately two hours. Through these contractions, the MMC gets rid of food particles in the small intestine and sends them to the large intestine. This only occurs during times of fasting, and it is completely shut down when we eat. In other words, the MMC only works when you are fasting. Spacing out your meals helps the MMC to function properly.

The MMC can easily become disrupted by consuming too many calories and not allowing three to four hours between meals. If you eat too often, there is no time to move food through the organs to the digestive system, so it can be broken down, the nutrients absorbed, and the waste eliminated. The MMC is stimulated three to four hours post meal in a fasted state. The wave of contractions occurs and our food is digested. If this process is continually disrupted, it can lead to constipation, bloating, acid reflux, cramping, irritable bowel syndrome (IBS), and SIBO. Considering that most women north of 40 begin to experience digestive issues, dysregulation of the MMC is something we want to avoid.

Another benefit to intermittent fasting related to the microbiome in the gut is an improvement to mood. Serotonin is a hormone which affects our mood. It is produced mostly in the cells that line our gut, and these are cells produced by fasting. Depression affects more women than men and increases during midlife. Some research has indicated that intermittent fasting can decrease signs of depression.

Intermittent fasting helps to turn white fat into brown fat. There are three types of fat tissue in the body—brown, beige, and white. Brown fat is rich in mitochondria, the powerhouses of our cells. Brown fat produces heat to maintain our body temperature in cold conditions. Brown fat contains many more mitochondria (the cell powerhouse) than does white fat. These mitochondria burn calories to produce energy for heat. They appear to be able to use body fat for fuel. Beige fat also contains mitochondria and is able to burn rather than store calories. Beige fat is found beneath the skin near the collarbone and along the spine. On the other hand, white fat stores energy. White fat makes up the majority of body fat in adults. It's made up of large fat droplets (lipids) and is metabolically inactive (does not burn energy). It has been described as a storage space for the excess calories we consume.

Brown fat is not common in adults. It's found primarily in infants. However, recent research has found that we can turn our white fat into brown fat. Intermittent fasting can help with this process. In experiments with mice, one group was put on an every-day fasting pattern. The other group was permitted to eat whatever and whenever they wanted. It was found that the gut bacteria changed in the fasting group of mice causing the production of short-chain fatty acids from the gut. This, in turn, caused the white fat cells to turn into brown fat cells. Obesity and insulin resistance (leading to diabetes) were reversed.

We are not mice. However, mice do have a metabolism similar to that of humans. The findings of this experiment have the potential to unlock some exciting possibilities with intermittent fasting.

Intermittent fasting improves mitochondrial health. Mitochondria create 90 percent of the energy the body needs to function. They are the powerhouses of the cells that convert nutrients from food into energy and process oxygen. If they fail to produce energy, disease can occur, affecting the brain, heart, liver, kidneys, pancreas, nerves, pancreas, eyes, and ears.

Fasting can create new mitochondria by stimulating pathways, which build mitochondria through an enzyme called 5' adenosine monophosphate-activated protein kinase (AMPK). AMPK regulates energy metabolism and fat burning. It is believed that AMPK activity decreases as we age, causing changes in body weight and energy. AMPK activity increases with fasting.

Fasting also increases a family of proteins that allow your cells to work efficiently. These proteins are called sirtuins, and they regulate the metabolism of blood glucose (sugar), fight inflammation, and repair damage to the genetic matter in cells. They also increase energy levels and create new mitochondria. Sirtuins work with NAD+, a molecule that supplies the energy needed for sirtuins to function properly. NAD+ declines as we age, causing brain fog and decreased energy. It is improved by intermittent fasting.

Intermittent fasting supports mitochondrial uncoupling. When mitochondria start to get overly crowded with charged particles, some of them burst out to reduce the tension. A cell will make new mitochondria to accommodate all of the particles trying to couple. Your body requires fat stores, ketones, and certain proteins to make this happen. These proteins are called uncoupling proteins. They make it possible for uncoupled protons to leave mitochondria, and in the process of doing so, waste calories are also evacuated. Any process where electrons and protons leave the mitochondria without making energy is called mitochondrial uncoupling.

Mitochondrial uncoupling has many benefits, including:

- The "wasting of calories." This is a term used by Dr. Steven Gundry, former heart surgeon, cardiologist, and founder of the International Heart and Lung Institute. The term means more calories are expended, making it easier to lose and maintain weight.
- Protection of mitochondrial health and prevention of damage
- Production of heat through thermogenesis, which supports weight loss and good health

Intermittent fasting where calories are restricted for more than 12 hours at a time is linked to mitochondrial uncoupling. When this is combined with polyphenol-rich foods found in plants, our bodies have a natural ability to protect cells against oxidative stress. Oxidative stress is an imbalance of harmful free radicals and antioxidants in the body, which can lead to a breakdown in cell tissue and DNA damage resulting in inflammation. Inflammation is a precursor to chronic disease. Polyphenol-rich foods include cocoa powder, dark chocolate, cloves, blackberries, blueberries, pomegranates, raspberries, walnuts, pecans, artichokes, red onions, spinach, and green tea.

Intermittent fasting causes a process called autophagy, which was discovered in the 1970s by a Belgian scientist named Christian de Duve. Autophagy is a process where the body cleanses cells by getting rid of damaged, aging cells. Basically, your body "takes out the trash." It makes your cells cleaner and stronger.

During autophagy, your cells break down parts of themselves and place them in small cavities within the cells where they will be digested. The waste generated by the cells must be disposed of or it will become toxic to the cells, causing aging, hormonal imbalance, and loss of energy.

When you fast, autophagy speeds up after 24 to 48 hours and causes a state of ketosis. Ketosis is a state where fatty acids are used by the body as energy rather than glucose (sugar). Ketosis results in ketones, which will be your body's main source of fuel. At approximately 12 hours of fasting, your body will begin to enter ketosis and tap into its fat stores rather than using carbohydrates as energy.

The benefits of autophagy include the following:

- Anti-aging
- Improvements in skin
- A strengthening of the immune system by clearing out viruses and bacteria
- Prevention of dementia and Alzheimer's disease
- Reduction in inflammation, which causes autoimmune disease and potentially cancer

- Repair of damaged DNA, which can protect against cancer
- Improvement in metabolic health by protecting the health of the mitochondria

Intermittent fasting can improve the immune system by helping the body to clean out the digestive system and eliminate harmful microorganisms from the gut. It also allows the body uninterrupted time to rest and heal. If our bodies are working hard to digest food, we do not have the energy needed to heal.

Fasting kills old, damaged cells and creates new ones. It helps you to be more resistant to cellular toxins. It can also improve the regeneration of stem cells. Reduced stem cell function accelerates the aging process. In addition, fasting can reduce the release of cytokines, which are inflammatory proteins which can damage organs.

Improvement in brain health is one of the most exciting benefits to intermittent fasting. In my late forties, I began to notice an increase in brain fog and "fuzzy" thinking. A decrease in the brain hormone called brain-derived neurotrophic factor (BDNF) can cause depression, mood issues, and brain fog. BDNF declines with age and with the loss of estrogen as we approach menopause.

Beta-hydroxybutyrate (BHB) is a ketone that helps your brain grow new brain cells and make new connections between them. It protects the brain against neurodegenerative disorders. BHB is produced more quickly by fasting and a low-carbohydrate diet. Too much glucose (blood sugar) is toxic to the brain. Ketones and BHB are a better fuel source for cognition than glucose.

Fasting also clears out beta-amyloid plaques, which are believed to be associated with dementia and damage to brain tissue. It protects against neurodegeneration.

Stage of Life Considerations

There is no one best health plan that fits every woman. As a woman, you need to consider your stage of life—whether or not you are cycling, in perimenopause, in menopause, or beyond. Each life stage requires a different approach to intermittent fasting, as well as nutrition and exercise. Before we look at intermittent fasting and how it plays out with the stages of life, let's review the stages of life: cycling, in perimenopause, in menopause, and beyond.

When You're Cycling

When you are cycling, you will go through hormonal fluctuations. Your cortisol levels will shift and your metabolism may change. Body temperature, glucose levels, sleep quality, and energy will fluctuate during each phase. This is caused by your internal menstrual clock, which occurs over a 28-day menstrual cycle. This is referred to as the infradian rhythm, and it consists of these phases:

- Phase 1: Follicular
- Phase 2: Ovulatory
- Phase 3: Luteal
- Ending in menstruation

The Follicular Phase

In this phase your body prepares itself to receive a fertilized egg for implantation in the uterus. At the beginning of this phase, estrogen levels are low and gradually increase as you move closer to ovulation.

When estrogen decreases, it causes the release of follicle-stimulating hormone (FSH), which prompts the ovaries to create follicles where estrogen is produced. Each follicle contains a mature egg. The healthiest egg remains while the rest of the follicles are reabsorbed into the body. Once this occurs your body will release extra estrogen.

The follicular phase is usually days six to 14 of your cycle and concludes when you ovulate. During this time, estrogen fluctuates and may be too low or too high. This can cause low cortisol and slower metabolism or higher energy and better moods, depending on the levels. When estrogen is higher, glucose levels are lower, and you are naturally more insulin sensitive.

During the follicular phase, you should:

- Eat phytoestrogen-containing foods such as flaxseeds, berries, and chickpeas that will support healthy levels of estrogen.
- Include fermented foods such as cabbage, carrots, and cucumbers that create diversity in the microbiome.
- Increase foods with omega-3 fatty acids such as salmon in order to decrease inflammation.
- Eat non-starchy vegetables and non-processed starch such as sweet potatoes or winter squash.

The Ovulatory Phase

This phase occurs between days 15 to 17 of your cycle and begins when the ovary releases a mature egg for a possible pregnancy. You will most likely feel a higher sex drive, increased energy, and a sense of wellbeing and confidence.

During this phase, it's recommended you do the following:

- Emphasize quality protein, which helps your body build, repair, and maintain muscle and keeps you feeling full and satiated.
- Concentrate on getting enough vitamin B and vitamin C. Vitamin B keeps you calm and protects

the nervous system. Vitamin C helps control stress and boosts collagen, which supports skin and joints. Vitamin B is found in quality grass-fed and organic animal proteins. Vitamin C is abundant in fruit and leafy greens.

- Consume healthy fats in the form of olive oil, avocados, nuts, and seeds. These will help you meet the high energy demands of ovulation.
- Don't forget about the liver. The liver is responsible for detoxification. The liver loves beets, garlic, cruciferous vegetables, dandelion greens, and artichokes.

The Luteal Phase

The luteal phase is marked by a rapid decline in estrogen, FSH, and LH and occurs from days 18 to 28 of your cycle. The follicle turns into a mass of cells called the corpus luteum, which secretes large amounts of progesterone. If the egg is not fertilized, the corpus luteum dissolves into the body, and both estrogen and progesterone drop. The uterine lining will be disposed of through the menstrual flow. You then enter the one to five days of menstruation.

When estrogen and progesterone get out of balance, this causes PMS symptoms to occur. During this phase, you may feel hungrier, be moody, less energetic, and experience food cravings. Glucose (blood sugar) can increase, making you less sensitive to insulin.

To avoid PMS, do the following:

- Because you are potentially insulin resistant, avoid processed carbohydrates, sugary foods, dairy, and alcohol.
- Focus on omega-3 fatty acids from fatty fish to control inflammation.

- Emphasize vitamin B, magnesium (spinach, nuts, seeds), and selenium (Brazil nuts).
- Avoid high sodium to prevent bloating.
- Stay away from gluten, which is inflammatory.

The Menstruation Phase

At this time, the lining of the uterus will be shed, creating bleeding. Both estrogen and progesterone are low. Energy is decreased and the mood tends to be low.

It is recommended in this phase that you focus on the following:

- Consume bone broth, which can provide collagen and protein.
- Drink herbal teas such as dandelion to relieve symptoms of PMS.
- Avoid gluten, and choose sweet potatoes and brown rice instead.
- Add beets for circulation and energy.
- Eat foods high in phytoestrogens such as colorful plants. These will also help reduce inflammation and pain and protect your body from free radicals.
- Consume mushrooms, which fight inflammation.
- Limit caffeine, and avoid alcohol, excess salt, and bad fats (such as greasy fast food).
- Eat enough high-quality protein.

How to Intermittent Fast During Cycling

Follow these guidelines for intermittent fasting during cycling:

- The first three weeks of your cycle are the best time to fast if you are on a regular 28-day cycle because your hormones are more stable. You can take advantage of this time to decrease inflammation and insulin.

- You may need to avoid fasting during the five to seven days preceding your cycle because you need to support your hormones with additional nutrients during the luteal phase.
- Be aware of your stress levels. You should not fast when you are under high amounts of stress because fasting increases cortisol levels, which can cause an imbalance in estrogen and progesterone.
- Do not restrict calories. Focus on quality nutrition during your feeding window.
- If you have PCOS, fasting 12 to 16 hours can be beneficial in balancing insulin and supporting weight loss.
- If you are planning on getting pregnant, avoid fasting. You will need an adequate energy supply and nutrients from stored fat and food to support a healthy pregnancy.
- You will need to keep your fasting schedule flexible when you are under the age of 35 in order to support your menstrual cycle. This schedule would be every other day or a few days per week. Women over 40 can usually do a more regular fasting window.
- Your blood glucose (sugar levels) needs to be balanced. Concentrate on meals that prioritize protein and healthy fats.

Perimenopause

Perimenopause is a window of time where the sex hormones begin to fluctuate and eventually decline as we transition into menopause. Symptoms typically begin in the early forties but can start as early as our mid- to late thirties. However, every woman is different. It has been described as being much like puberty. The difference is that our sex hormones are declining rather than increasing.

As progesterone declines, our body no longer releases an egg each month, and cycles become irregular. Levels of the stress hormone cortisol tend to rise and can make us more vulnerable to stress. We become more likely to be insulin resistant. Sleep can be disrupted because less melatonin is released.

Levels of estrogen can rise at the beginning of perimenopause because of lower progesterone. Estrogen and progesterone fluctuate like a seesaw. One hormone will be higher, and the other will be lower.

Perimenopause symptoms can include hot flashes, night sweats, moodiness, change in libido, irregular ovulation and menstruation, and sleep problems. Many women find this time to be more difficult than menopause.

Perimenopause can also result in loss of bone and cardiovascular issues because of the loss of estrogen. The risk of osteoporosis increases after perimenopause, and you can gradually lose bone more quickly than your body can replace it. The risk of heart disease also increases due to declining estrogen. This is where intermittent fasting can help. A 2019 study published in *Circulation* found that people who do intermittent fasting were 70 percent less likely to suffer from heart failure than those who had never fasted. There have also been studies that suggest risks for insulin resistance, metabolic inflexibility, and inflammation were reduced by fasting.

If you are intermittent fasting, be sure you are getting enough sleep, balancing stress, and sustaining a nutritious diet. If you are under high amounts of stress, you may want to wait to incorporate intermittent fasting. Fasting can be a good form of stress for your body. However, cortisol does increase, which lowers progesterone and estrogen. As already mentioned, if you are still cycling, the first 21 days are usually the best time to fast.

My experience with perimenopause was much like a rollercoaster. Looking back, I can see that my symptoms began at about age 37. My periods became extremely heavy, and I developed fibroids. This was most likely due to decreased progesterone levels and increased estrogen, causing estrogen dominance. At age 40, one fibroid became so large that my gynecologist suggested I have a partial hysterectomy. I consented, believing I had no other alternatives.

My uterus was removed, but my ovaries were left intact. My doctor told me that leaving my ovaries would ensure I would not go into early menopause. Nothing could have prepared me for the symptoms I experienced over the next 10 years. I later learned that having my uterus removed put me at an increased risk of ovarian failure, which in turn affected my estrogen levels. All progesterone was depleted from my body. I had lost the hormone that gives a sense of wellbeing and calm. This accelerated and intensified many of the perimenopausal symptoms, such as poor sleep, anxiety, and night sweats. In addition, I went through all the hormonal stages of perimenopause but without the monthly bleeding. This was confusing for me because it seemed physical symptoms were unpredictable without a monthly cycle to gauge where I was in the process. My doctor did not prepare me. Rather, he made it seem as if surgery would easily resolve the physical symptoms I was experiencing. Yes, it resolved the excessive bleeding, but it created an entire host of hormonal problems.

I reached out to my gynecologist numerous times only to be told my estrogen levels were within normal range. Looking back, I realize my estrogen levels were on the low end of normal. Progesterone was never once mentioned. I would later learn that doctors considered this hormone unnecessary if you did not have a uterus. I had no idea that my body was missing the benefits of progesterone for anxiety and sleep.

By the time I reached age 48, the hot flashes, night sweats, and sleep problems were profound. What I didn't understand at the time was that estrogen levels were falling, estradiol was low, and my blood sugar was most likely fluctuating. An understanding of my body and hormonal balance would have helped me make better decisions. I would have asked my doctor more questions and most likely would have opted against having a hysterectomy. I would have understood the perimenopausal symptoms and honored my body by getting quality sleep, good nutrition, and not over-exercising. I would not have taken my hormones for granted.

I was also beginning to experience gut issues and food sensitivities. My stomach pain was so acute that I sought the help of a gastroenterologist who eventually diagnosed me with irritable bowel syndrome (IBS). I believe this was potentially the beginning of my road to autoimmune disease and led to my development of rheumatoid disease and thyroid malfunction.

One of the greatest symptoms I experienced in perimenopause was mood changes. I struggled with depression and anxiety. At times, my patience was short because of irritability. I had lost progesterone, estrogen was declining, sleep was poor, and I was feeling the stress of caring for two generations. I was caring for three young children at the same time as I was caring for my aging parents. This is often referred to as the "sandwich generation."

The most difficult moment in my forties came the year my parents died within six months of each other. My mother passed suddenly two days before Thanksgiving from heart failure. At the time, I was caring for both my father who had come to live with us after his diagnosis of cancer and my three young children, ages 10, eight, and six years.

I recall a day when hospice was delivering a hospital bed for my ailing father. My oldest daughter had disappeared into her bedroom with her friend. When she emerged, her bangs had been completely cut off to the scalp. She had a big smile on her face, and her friend was standing beside her holding a pair of household scissors. At that moment, I burst into tears. The tears were not the result of disappointment with my daughter. The tears were the result of feeling overwhelmed.

During the perimenopausal years, it's important to have a stress management plan that includes self-care. Stress keeps us in a continual fight-or-flight state that elevates cortisol and eventually impacts our health. This can cause weight gain, problems with insulin regulation, and a compromised immune system. Here are a few steps you can take to manage stress:

- Have a morning routine. How you start your day determines the quality of your life.
- Expose yourself to sunshine for a few minutes in the morning. Vitamin D from sunshine is a stress reliever because it helps your body to produce serotonin, which can improve your mood and help you to stay calm.
- Keep a gratitude journal where you write down one to three things each day that you are thankful to have in your life. These need not be complex. (I recently wrote that I was thankful for the cup of coffee my husband brought me in the morning.)
- Incorporate both exercise and daily movement into your life. Movement can include exercise. However, it also includes all of your non-exercise activities such as gardening, walking the dog, or

cleaning the house. Finding a way to move daily can be beneficial for overall health and wellbeing.

Set boundaries with yourself and others. As women we continually allow stress to rule our days and rob us of joy and peace. Overwhelming yourself with work, events, and requests will create stress. Say yes to the projects that benefit your mind, body, and soul, and no to the ones which drain your energy. Let your "no" stand alone. There's no need to explain your reasons to anyone.

Make time for learning. This can include anything from an educational health podcast to a book on self-improvement. I listen to an inspirational podcast daily. The topics vary from health and fitness to science, business, and self-help. This does not include listening to or watching current world events or politics. This should be something that encourages you to learn and grow as a woman. Be a lifelong learner.

Have a nighttime routine. Think of your morning and nighttime routines as bookends for your days. Ending the day on a positive note will allow for better sleep and prevent a cortisol-awakening response.

- Dim the lights in your home.
- Silence and set aside your phone and all electronics at least 60 minutes prior to bedtime. Because I run an online business, eliminating nighttime electronics is something I'm consciously and continually working towards.
- Read a book or your gratitude journal. Reflect on all the people for whom you are thankful.
- Consider prayer, deep breathing, or meditation to calm your brain.
- Give yourself three to four hours between dinner and bedtime. This allows time for your body to

digest and rest and will support your circadian rhythms. If you eat too close to bedtime, you release glucose and elevate cortisol levels, making it difficult to go into deep sleep.

- Take a hot shower or bath but have the bedroom cool so that you reap the benefits of hot and cold therapy. If you can stand cold water, end your shower this way. This helps induce sleep and regenerate hormones.

Have the room dark to encourage the secretion of melatonin.

Menopause

Menopause occurs when a woman has gone without a menstrual period for 12 consecutive months. Approximately 85 percent of women will experience symptoms such as hot flashes, night sweats, vaginal dryness, brain fog, mood swings, depression, and headaches.

Menopause requires shifts in how we exercise and eat. Eating high-quality protein becomes even more important because of the loss of estrogen leading to decreased muscle mass (sarcopenia). Strength training should be emphasized to prevent sarcopenia and bone loss.

Other things to consider with nutrition during menopause include the following:

- Eliminate gluten, which is highly inflammatory and can cause gut issues.
- Increase fruits and vegetables to minimize weight gain while increasing fiber, antioxidants, and nutrients. Prioritize non-starchy vegetables over fruits at a three-to-one ratio.

- Be sure you are getting enough calcium. Your calcium intake needs to increase during menopause because of the loss of estrogen, which can increase bone loss. Because dairy can be highly inflammatory, it's best to get calcium from non-dairy sources such as sardines, turnip greens, Bok choy, mustard greens, and other plant foods.
- Eat healthy fats from fish, avocados, coconut oil, olive oil, and nuts to support hormone balance. Omega-3 fatty acids from fish can help eliminate inflammation.
- Avoid processed foods and refined sugar, which can trigger hot flashes and contribute to weight gain.
- Pay close attention to your hydration needs. You should drink at least half of your body weight in ounces of water daily. Consider supplementing the water with electrolytes to allow your cells to communicate and perform basic functions. This is especially important if intermittent fasting when electrolytes can be flushed out of the body. The cells in your body need water and all metabolic processes use it. Dehydration causes the loss of elasticity in your skin and contributes to vaginal dryness.

One of the benefits of menopause and beyond is fewer restrictions surrounding intermittent fasting. You are no longer working around your menstrual cycle, and fasting can reduce symptoms such as hot flashes, fatigue, and brain fog. Intermittent fasting can slow the aging process by regenerating your cells and mitochondria.

Intermittent fasting is not a diet or weight loss plan. Rather, it is a lifestyle tool for creating metabolic flexibility, brain health, mental clarity, increased energy, and potentially a better healthspan. Perimenopause can bring major hormonal fluctuations in estrogen, progesterone, cortisol, and insulin. Crossing the threshold of menopause creates challenges as we experience more problems with regulating insulin and a loss of some key hormones. Intermittent fasting can bring hormones such as insulin in balance. One of the things that makes intermittent fasting more effective is the right type and amount of exercise. In the next chapter, we will explore the exercise that is best for women over the ages of 40 and 50.

Chapter 5

An Exercise Prescription for Midlife Women

A little over a year ago, Mary joined my Fit and Fierce program for women over 40. She was a 57-year-old avid long-distance runner who enjoyed long, challenging hikes on the weekend. Her goals were to tone up and reduce belly fat.

She was not overweight according to the body mass index (BMI). BMI is a body fat measurement, which uses height and weight. Because it doesn't take into account muscle or skeletal frame, it's not an accurate way to assess fitness levels. However, the starting photos and measurements revealed that Mary had a high amount of body fat, which was centered mostly in her waistline. In fact, her waist-to-hip ratio was 0.86, which is considered a high risk for cardiovascular disease according to the World Health Organization. Waist-to-hip ratio measures your waist circumference to your hip circumference and is thought to be a more accurate measure for health risks than BMI.

There were two main areas I addressed with Mary. First, I looked at nutrition and helped her calculate a balanced macro ratio. Second, I adjusted her weekly exercise training plan. I added three 30-minute strength training workouts per week and *reduced the amount of long, endurance-type cardio. I knew she enjoyed the hikes, and the "joy" factor is important, so I included one long hike per week. She reduced her running to two light jogs, and we added two short 15-minute high intensity interval training (HIIT) sessions.*

Within 12 weeks, Mary lost 14 pounds, increased her skeletal muscle, reduced her body fat by six percent, and reduced her waistline by 3.5 inches, bringing her waist-to-hip ratio down to 0.81. She even purchased a bikini to celebrate the changes she was seeing in her body.

Decreasing Mary's long endurance cardio to reduce body fat may seem counterintuitive. However, it is part of an overall strategy to increase muscle, reduce adipose tissue, and increase basal metabolic rate. As we move through this chapter, you will see that exercise is a prescription. Just like intermittent fasting, when done correctly, it can yield positive physical results.

For most of my life I was obsessed with cardio exercise, and this obsession reached a peak in my late forties. In my twenties, it was step aerobics and jazzercise. In the first half of my thirties, it was long 20-mile hikes in the New Mexico mountains. After we adopted our first child from China in my mid-thirties, I switched to studio cycling classes.

In my forties, I took it to the next level with marathons and century 100-mile bike rides. My first marathon was one week prior to a 110-mile biking event in the steep winding mountains of Taos and Red River.

From there, I participated in a quadrathlon on Mount Taylor. This entailed biking up to the base of the mountain, running several miles further, snowshoeing for the third quarter of the event, and cross-country skiing to the top.

From there we reversed the order of the activities all the way back down the mountain to the starting point. It was absolutely grueling.

In the second half of my forties, I concentrated solely on running as many marathons as I could, including two Boston Marathons. I became first regionally and then nationally ranked for my age division. At 47 I added in trail running and took first overall place in a local bosque run. As I began to concentrate on speed and shorter distances such as 10K and 5K events, I took up cardio boxing and boot camp classes. To say I was over-exercising would be an understatement. I was absolutely beating my body into the ground.

A typical week consisted of clocking 75 to 100 miles of running, four cardio boxing classes, two body pump classes, two boot camp classes, and one hot yoga vinyasa class. Monday would begin with an early morning run. I would get the kids off to school and drive to the gym for a cardio boxing class. Tuesday would be focused on a long run. Wednesday was running and cardio boxing in the morning and body pump and boot camp class in the evening. Thursday was a long run. Friday was running, boot camp, and cardio boxing. Saturday was running, cardio boxing, and body pump. Sunday was hot vinyasa yoga.

You get the picture. Rest and recovery were nowhere on the schedule. Strength training was limited to body pump classes, which focused more on endurance and the aerobic aspect of lifting weights.

Cracked ribs from a fall during a trail run, hip bursitis, a torn meniscus, and a back injury doing a burpee did not stop me. It would take a broken metatarsal and a ruptured plantar fascia to finally change the course of my exercise routine.

When I broke the metatarsal in my left foot, I was in a boot cast for eight weeks. I was out of the cast for one week when I ruptured my plantar fascia on my right foot while sprinting. This led to another eight weeks in a boot cast with three months of physical therapy to restore full function in my foot. During those five months of recovery, I began working with a personal trainer and lifting weights. The only reason I did strength training was because it was literally all I could do. I thought weight lifting was inferior. All I wanted to do was to get back to running.

Yet something happened in those 16 weeks. I began to notice muscle tone and definition in my shoulders and arms. People at the gym began complimenting me on my shoulders. I didn't feel as exhausted. This was a turning point in my health and fitness. I didn't yet have the nutrition and lifestyle pieces of the puzzle, but I was beginning to see positive changes in my body. It would be another two years before I finally gave up running and learned the power of nutrition, but I had changed the trajectory of my life.

When we go through perimenopause and ultimately menopause, we need a different approach to exercise. What worked in our twenties and thirties no longer serves us in our forties, fifties, and beyond. I didn't understand this and ultimately caused damage with a poor diet, little sleep, high stress, and over-exercising. I believe these lifestyle habits led to my developing autoimmune disease.

My goal now is to educate women on the lifestyle habits that affect our hormones and ultimately our health and longevity. I don't want to see other women endure the suffering I experienced in my mid- to late forties. Menopause is a normal part of life. However, the choices we make can determine whether we crash into menopause or transition with grace and ease.

In this chapter you will learn how exercise can help you live a longer life, how to train according to your natural bodily rhythms, the exercise mistakes to avoid, the best type of exercise to tone muscles and burn fat, and how to avoid exercise burnout.

Longevity and Quality of Life

You may have heard that results are based on 80 percent nutrition and 20 percent exercise. Even though I am a proponent of quality whole-food nutrition, I disagree with this statement. Research is consistently indicating that exercise is one of the best predictors for reducing all causes of mortality as we age. Yes, nutrition is key to seeing that hidden six pack in your abs. However, when it comes to quality and potentially quantity of life, exercise is extremely powerful.

According to Dr. Ben Bickman, it is believed that Alzheimer's may be partially attributed to brain insulin resistance. When the brain becomes insulin resistant, it cannot get as much energy. Thus, it goes hungry. A recent paper cited a study, which shows that an eight-week exercise intervention program in sedentary individuals can restore insulin action in the brain, reversing some brain insulin resistance. The individuals who exercised for eight weeks experienced improved cognition.

There is something that happens in strength and activity level with age. Both drastically drop, especially past the age of 75. Exercise is a way to preserve strength as we move through the decades. The sooner we start, the better the outcome in later years. Even light exercise carries a benefit.

A recent study found that individuals who exercised two to four times more than the American Heart Association's weekly minimum recommendation of 150 minutes of moderate activity had a reduction in mortality risk of 26 percent to 31 percent.

Over a 30-year period, the National Institutes of Health did a peer reviewed study that analyzed the activity of 100,000 adults. They found that meeting the activity guidelines of 150 minutes of moderate exercise weekly also had significant but lower benefits. Those individuals had a reduction in mortality risk of 20 percent to 21 percent. Vigorous exercise for 75 minutes had a 19 percent reduction in mortality risk.

Another study looked at 8,000 Canadians between the ages of 65 to 86. Researchers looked at problem solving, attention, working memory, and organizational skills. They found that lower muscle mass may be associated with steeper cognitive decline in age.

Studies have also determined that there is a correlation between leg strength and brain function at age 80. To maintain strength, it's important that we do more than exercise. To show up fully and have the strength to exercise, we, as women, must prioritize sleep and protect our brain health. Proper nutrition is essential. However, we must also avoid the things which lead to poor gut and brain health, such as sugar, inflammatory foods, and alcohol abuse.

The bottom line is exercise can potentially improve how we age. In perimenopause and menopause, we still need to be cognizant of matching our training to our hormones, energy, and stress levels. However, there is congruence in most studies showing the overall benefits of exercise at each and every stage of life. We just need to be willing to embrace those benefits.

Periodization

It can be beneficial to structure our exercise routine around a specific cycle or time period. This is often referred to as periodization. Periodization is where various training variables such as frequency, load, and volume are manipulated in order to optimize performance, make ongoing progress, and avoid overtraining and injury. Training intensity is varied over a set period of time.

Periodization is a technique frequently used by athletes and one I used when training for marathons. I had weeks where I advanced in miles and speed and weeks where I backed off the intensity. The goal was to increase my endurance and speed without increasing the likelihood of an injury.

This same method can be effective for midlife women. It can be centered around a woman's monthly 28-day cycle or around the lunar cycle if a woman has gone through menopause. This will be in alignment with natural circadian rhythms. Keep in mind that the schedule may need to be altered if a woman has irregular cycles such as in perimenopause.

Let's unpack what a periodization cycle might entail. In this model, week one is the menstruation cycle rather than week four.

Week 1—Menstruation or the New Moon

This begins on the first day of menstruation and continues for one week. Menopausal women will follow the new moon phase. During this time, estrogen and progesterone are low. Fatigue is high. You will want to give yourself 48 to 72 hours between strength training sessions.

Moderate weights are recommended with a repetition range of 10 to 15. Please note that the total volume of sets and reps is bio-individual and based on many different factors, such as stage of life, sleep, energy, overall health, fitness level, and goals. If you are just starting out, do two sets of 10 to 15 repetitions, use lighter weights, and keep the workout at no more than 30 minutes. If you are a more experienced lifter, aim for three to four sets for a total of 45 to 60 minutes.

Include moderate daily exercise, such as walking, and some restorative activities, such as gentle yoga, stretching, meditation, and prayer.

Week 2—Ovulation or First Quarter of the Lunar Cycle

During ovulation, testosterone and estrogen peak. Ligaments have more laxity due to increased estrogen. Focus on building muscle with heavier weights and a lower rep range of 10 or less. Again, this is bio-individual. If you are new to strength training, keep sessions at 30 minutes, do fewer sets, and use lighter weights. Take 48 hours before training the same muscle group. For example, if you train shoulders on Monday, wait until Wednesday to train them again. If you are very sore, allow 72 hours of recovery. Remember, every woman is unique and will require a different rest period.

Because ligaments are lax, high impact HIIT (high intensity interval training) should be avoided. Aim for lower impact cardio exercise, such as cycling, elliptical, walking, swimming, and rowing, three days this week.

Week 3—The Luteal Phase 1 or the Full Moon

Estrogen is typically high. Progesterone will peak at approximately day 21. HIIT can be intense but should still be lower impact. If you are accustomed to HIIT, incorporate three 15-minute sessions this week (not including warm up and cool down). Strength training should be done with moderate weight. Again, adjust sets, reps, time, and weight for your level of fitness.

Week 4—The Luteal Phase 2 or Last Quarter of the Lunar Cycle

Progesterone declines. Consider doing shorter, less intense HIIT sessions and focusing on muscular endurance with higher repetition weight lifting. I sometimes give clients

10-minute HIIT workouts after strength training sessions. Reps should be in the 15 to 20 range. Allow 48 to 72 hours before training the same body part. If you are new to weight training, you may want to do only one to two sets per exercise because of the increased repetition range. It can also be helpful to engage in less intense activities such as:

- Pilates
- Yoga
- Walking
- Cross training with a different mode of cardio, such as elliptical, stationary bike, hiking, or swimming

Once we transition fully into menopause, we do not need to be tied to certain types of exercise and particular times of the month. However, because research indicates that women over 50 benefit from having more recovery, the periodization cycle can be helpful. As a general rule, allow 48 to 72 hours before training the same body part. If you do legs on Tuesday, you won't train legs again until Thursday or Friday. If you do full body workouts, aim for two to three per week with adequate rest between the sessions.

How Much and What Type of Exercise

I typically give my clients anywhere from two to four strength training days per week, two to three short HIIT sessions per week, and three to four lower impact activities such as walking, hiking, swimming, or yoga. As I mentioned before, specific exercise plans are bio-individual and based on many lifestyle factors as well as the client's fitness level and health goals. I have found with myself and working with clients that daily movement of some type is highly beneficial. Once women are in perimenopause and beyond, it's beneficial to moderate exercise intensity. You need to move daily, but you don't want every day to be packed with the type of exercise intensity you would experience in a boot camp.

For example, I have a client named Susan who is 53 and has transitioned into menopause. Before I create a custom training program for a client, I do an intake where I ask a series of questions covering sleep, energy, hormonal symptoms, signs of cortisol dysregulation, and their desired outcome. Susan's goals are to increase skeletal muscle, decrease body fat, and fit into a dress she wants to wear at her daughter's wedding. Her energy and sleep quality are good, and she is working with a functional medicine doctor to balance her hormone levels. Susan has been strength training for over a year and has built up to a healthy fitness level. Here is the plan she is following:

Day 1—30 minutes of a lower body (legs and glutes) strength training workout, which includes squats, lunges, step ups, the leg press, and a hip hinge exercise such as a deadlift or glute hip thrust.

Day 2—30 minutes of zone 2 cardio of her choice (walking, jogging, stair stepper, rower, etc.). Zone 2 cardio is a moderate level just below endurance. You are able to talk between breaths to someone, but they would know you are exercising by your breath. Zone 2 cardio is something you could conceivably maintain for a long period of time. She can use her Fitbit or level of perceived exertion to monitor her effort.

Day 3—20 minutes of HIIT cardio of her choice (not including the warm up and cool down). If Susan has any sign of cortisol dysregulation, such as poor sleep or low energy, I would omit the HIIT cardio to reduce physical stress.

Day 4—30 minutes of upper body strength training, which includes a chest press, assisted pull-ups, seated rows, a shoulder press, and isolation exercises for the triceps and biceps. This is followed by 10 minutes of HIIT cardio.

Day 5—60 minutes of zone 2 cardio.

One restorative yoga session per week.

Please note that these days do not need to fall on any particular day of the week. She will choose the days that work within her schedule. Also, it's important to understand that there is no one way to structure an exercise program that is right for every midlife woman.

The key is to make those strength training days truly count. This means lifting heavy enough to stimulate muscle synthesis. If past nagging injuries prevent you from lifting heavier weights as it does with my back problems, there are numerous ways to still bring intensity to your exercise. You can increase repetitions or sets, decrease rest time, or use a technique called time under tension. Time under tension can involve slowing the reps down, actively squeezing and contracting the muscles while performing the reps, and using isometric holds at the peak contraction.

There is an ongoing debate on high versus low repetitions when weight lifting. You don't simply want to get tired after a strength training session. You want to lift to muscular fatigue. This is different from simply exhausting yourself. Performing endless repetitions with light weight won't do much to change your body. It will make you tired and potentially cause injury. You should feel the fatigue in the muscle group you are working and the last three repetitions should be difficult.

For example, if you are performing 15 reps of an overhead dumbbell shoulder press, the last three reps of each set should be challenging. It should also have a cumulative effect. If you are performing three sets, each set should be more difficult to complete than the last. The same principle applies whether you are doing 10, 12, or 20 reps of an exercise.

If you are a beginner, start slow. Concentrate on form. Hire a trainer who has experience working with midlife women. Start with only two sets, and work up to more. The intensity should not be added until you have mastered the form.

Progressive overload is an important part of muscle synthesis. If we lift with the same intensity each and every workout, we cease to progress. It's easier to maintain than it is to progress. There are ways to increase the intensity safely even if you have physical limitations. Here are a few of my favorite techniques for dialing up the intensity:

- *Supersets*: combine two exercises of opposing or the same muscle group. Perform each without stopping. Rest and repeat the remaining sets. For example, you can superset opposing muscle groups with a bicep curl and a tricep extension for 15 reps of each. Perform both exercises without stopping. Rest 60 seconds before doing the next set. I also like supersetting two exercises for the same muscle group. For example, you can perform a chest press with a chest fly for three sets of 12 reps.
- *Tri-sets*: this is the same concept as a superset, but you combine three exercises instead of two.
- *Giant sets*: this is again the same concept as supersets, but you are combining four to five exercises. This works well with shoulders and legs. For example, you could perform a shoulder press, lateral raise, front raise, rear delt fly, and an upright row. If you are new to strength training, perform the giant set one time. If you are at an intermediate

level of weight training, aim for three sets. A more experienced exerciser can do anywhere from three to five sets with up to two minutes of rest between the sets.

- *Drop sets*: this is one of my favorite training techniques. This involves moving from heavier to lighter weight. For example, perform 10 shoulder presses with your heaviest weight. Immediately pick up a slightly lighter weight and perform 10 more reps. Without stopping, pick up a lighter weight and perform the final 10 reps. I like to do a drop set for my final set of an exercise. Using the example above, you would perform three sets of 12 reps, resting 45 seconds between sets. For the fourth and final set, you would do a drop set of 10, 10, and 10, moving from your heaviest weight to your lightest weight without resting.

- *Pyramids*: pyramids add variety and intensity to your weight lifting routine. You can either pyramid down in weight or up in weight. Unlike drop sets, you will rest in between the sets. For example, do 15 leg presses. Rest 45 to 60 seconds. Increase weight and perform 12 reps. Rest. Increase weight, and perform 10 reps. Rest. Increase weight, and perform eight reps.

- *Finisher or burn-out sets*: these are an advanced training technique and are typically done as the last set of an exercise. They work well on isolation movements involving one muscle group, such as shoulders, biceps, or triceps. A burn-out set can be a drop set, or it can be a final set of an exercise, which goes to failure. (Be careful of form when doing this.) Failure means you perform as many reps as you can until you cannot perform another one with good

99

form. Failure does not mean continuing on with poor form and sustaining an injury as a result. An example of a failure set would be performing four sets of lateral raises with the fourth and final set going to failure (as many repetitions as you can).

- *Circuits*: circuits involve several different exercises. They can combine both upper and lower body exercises. Sometimes they include cardio such as jump rope. However, I advise against combining cardio with lifting. You will naturally receive some cardiovascular benefit when you work larger muscles such as the back or legs. However, I would steer clear of turning your lifting sessions into aerobic training. A good circuit would have three to four upper body exercises and three to four lower body exercises. You perform all the movements without stopping. Rest between rounds.

Full Body vs. Split Workouts

There are advantages and disadvantages to both full body versus split training styles. I believe the mode of training should be in alignment with your goals. For example, when I'm training for a bodybuilding competition, split training is best for me. Split training involves training certain muscle groups on certain days.

For split training, you would have a schedule, which might look like this: shoulders are worked on day one, legs are done on day two, chest and triceps are trained on day three, and finally, pull muscles (back and biceps) are completed on day four. There may even be a second leg day added. This is a great method to ensure each and every muscle group is developed. However, it is time-consuming and, in some cases, will not produce the largest metabolic benefit. It also does not allow for much rest time between training sessions.

Full body workouts are typically done two to three days per week and include primarily compound exercises, which work more than one muscle group and use multiple joints. This is a time-effective training schedule for busy women. It allows adequate rest time. It also uses more metabolic energy. However, it can be difficult to cover all the muscle groups (especially in two days of training). It also will not develop muscles such as glutes and shoulders to the full extent as does split training.

The important thing is to choose the mode of training that works with your schedule and that will help you meet your body goals. Be realistic with yourself as far as the time commitment and where you wish to train. If training from home with limited equipment, a full body workout may be a better option.

Compound vs. Isolation Exercises

For midlife women trying to reduce body fat and build muscle, compound movements will reap the highest benefit. Compound exercises are those that use multiple muscle groups, such as squats, lunges, leg presses, deadlifts, chest presses, and overhead shoulder presses. When I'm designing workouts for women, I typically use mostly compound movements.

Isolation exercises are those that only involve one muscle group, such as biceps, triceps, or the individual heads of the deltoid (front, side, rear). They have a place in defining and sculpting the body. However, many compound exercises will target those muscle groups as well. For example, a bent-over row also uses the biceps. A shoulder press can include chest and triceps muscles.

I typically sprinkle in isolation moves after the compound exercises. For example, chest and back exercises could be followed by bicep or tricep movements. Squats and lunges could be followed by glute kickbacks to isolate the glute muscles.

Common Mistakes

There are a few common exercise mistakes that I see women over 40 continually make. There is no judgment here. Trust me when I say that I made every mistake possible with my nutrition, exercise, and lifestyle choices in my forties. Awareness and education are vital and empowering.

Mistake 1: Over-Exercising

This was one that took me decades to learn. When we are in our twenties and thirties, we are more resilient. As we lose the protection of our hormones, we become more sensitive to stress and begin to experience issues with cortisol regulation.

Exercise is a good form of stress for our body if done correctly. However, when we do excessive amounts of cardio, we release cortisol. If that exercise is done in the evening or at night, this can disrupt sleep. Cortisol is typically highest in the morning and drops off in the late afternoon as we approach bedtime. However, if we do a 60-minute HIIT session at 6:00 p.m., we could cause elevated cortisol, making it difficult to fall asleep.

Although we need plenty of daily movement, strength training and some high intensity cardio and under-eating combined with excessive exercise can be detrimental to hormonal balance. I look back at photos of myself that were taken in the height of my running days. I look older in my forties than I do in my sixties!

I realize there is a joy factor to endurance exercise, so I will never say, "Don't run a marathon or do a triathlon." However, I will say to train smart and incorporate adequate rest and recovery into your weekly routine. This was the number one mistake I made. I thought I was invincible. My schedule had little recovery time, and I had the injuries to prove it.

The right amount of cardio, according to research, tends to include lots of zone 2 activities such as walking and hiking and a strategic amount of zone 5 activities in the form of intervals. Strength training is always a priority.

Mistake 2: Random Workouts With No Clear Objective or Plan

This is something I see all the time at the gym. Women will wander the gym doing a little of this and little of that. The order and grouping of the exercises matter. You should follow a clear, well-thought-out program designed specifically for you as a midlife woman, and it should be specific to your goals. Random workouts create random results.

Mistake 3: Following a YouTube Exercise Program That Is Designed to Look Cool but Yields No Results and May Cause Injury

This is another frequent issue I see. Social media fitness influencers are often more concerned with putting out a reel or YouTube video that is attention-grabbing than one that is well considered and safe. I get it. A trainer doing a dumbbell shoulder press isn't as impressive as balancing on an upside-down BOSU ball doing barbell deadlifts or clean and jerks (and yes, I've actually seen this).

When I taught group fitness, the goal of the classes was often to entertain. In fact, when I was going through my training, the instructor actually told me this. Trainers and fitness instructors are often in competition to create the hardest classes without thought to the safety or the efficacy for women over 40. I was guilty of this too. The pressure to fill classes was very real.

Mistake 4: Not Hiring a Trainer

I realize not everyone can afford a trainer. However, if you can purchase a few sessions to work on form and proper use of the equipment, it could spare you from injury. Having experienced eyes on your lifting technique will help you yield better physical results and potentially protect you from harm. This is especially true of exercises such as squats or deadlifts, which can cause a spinal injury.

I have two ruptured discs in my lower back that have caused, at times, debilitating pain. I believe much of this was brought on by not implementing proper technique in the beginning and by choosing exercises (such as burpees) that were not appropriate for my stage of life. I was oblivious to the harm I was causing until it was too late.

Mistake 5: Hiring the Wrong Trainer

It's not uncommon to see a woman over 50 working with a trainer who doesn't understand her unique needs. I see two mistakes made by trainers. First, younger trainers are often not properly trained on the hormonal changes associated with perimenopause and menopause. They give their 50-year-old female client the same exercise prescription as their 30-year-old clients. Secondly, some trainers assume that the workouts for a midlife woman should be easier because of age.

We need intensity in our fifties more than ever before. However, we need the right amount and type of intensity. For example, consider a woman who is 53 and struggling with excess body fat and muscle loss. She doesn't need to sit on one bicep curl machine for 10 minutes. She needs more compound exercises and supersets structured in a way that will yield the highest metabolic effect.

Mistake 6: Ignoring Your Body's Cues and Doing a Workout Just Because It's Part of Your Program

I'm a big believer in having a workout plan. However, there are times you will need to alter the plan because of stress, lack of sleep, or fatigue. When I was prepping for my last bodybuilding show, I followed a schedule for my strength training and cardio. Certain days called for HIIT (high intensity intervals). However, I have rheumatoid arthritis, an autoimmune disease that can cause joint pain and fatigue. When I felt I was on the edge of a flare up from overtraining, I would swap HIIT on the StairMaster for a walk on the treadmill.

Mistake 7: Doing More Cardio Than Strength Training

Cardio has its place for overall health. However, it's a poor weight-loss tool and can cause you to lose muscle when done incorrectly. When I was a marathon runner in my forties, I was bewildered. In my mind, running equaled being lean and toned. I thought running would give me beautiful legs and a flat stomach.

The opposite happened. My weight was low, but I had excess body fat on my lower belly and my legs lost all muscle. What I didn't realize at the time was that my body was rapidly losing muscle in those perimenopausal years. As I lost lean muscle mass, body fat increased and my skin began to sag. The result was thin, flabby legs and flat glutes.

I like to think of cardio as a prescription. You wouldn't take an entire bottle of antibiotics. You would only take what the doctor prescribed. The same is true of cardio. In the right dose, it will help. In extreme amounts, it places oxidative stress on your body, burns away muscle mass, and can make it even more difficult to lose weight. As explained earlier, oxidative stress is caused by an imbalance between free radicals and antioxidants in the body and can damage the DNA. It is associated with diseases such as diabetes, heart disease, cancer, and neurodegenerative conditions. I often describe over-exercising as aging at the cellular level.

When we have skeletal muscle, we have a more efficient metabolism. Muscle is a disposal site for glucose (blood sugar). According to a paper published by PubMed, healthy skeletal muscle is the largest "glucose sink" in the body. Seventy-five percent of glucose is disposed of through skeletal muscle. The first place we become insulin resistant is in the muscles. When we lose quality skeletal muscle, we lose our ability to regulate insulin.

Mistake 8: Not Using All the Pillars of Exercise

When exercising for fitness, health, longevity, and quality of life, we need to consider more than just one factor. Our weekly exercise plan should include stability, strength, zone 2 training, and zone 5 training.

Stability includes learning the proper movement patterns of exercises, such as squats and deadlifts, to avoid injury. If we approach strength training simply by how much weight we can lift or move, we may be doing so at the risk of sacrificing form. We want to move in a way that increases trunk stability and hip strength.

In order to change body composition and shape, we need strength training. However, resistance training is about more than aesthetics and how we look in a bikini. It's about living a long and healthy life. It's about being able to take the stairs in our later years or play with our grandkids and great-grandkids.

We also need a significant amount of zone 2 training. This is a level you can maintain for a period of time. For example, you're hiking but still able to maintain a conversation. It is a level just below your aerobic threshold. You are working above the easy zone but not pushing too hard. Ideally it should account for about three hours per week of your overall training. Beginners should aim for two hours of training in the zone 2 level. I do about four zone 2 workouts per week.

Zone 5 is the highest intensity level and should account for the least amount of your overall activity. I typically do two to three short HIIT (high intensity interval training) sessions per week. On average I do a total of 20 to 30 minutes per week. This could be two 15-minute sessions or three 10-minute ones. The length of these sessions varies for me and my clients. I look at sleep quality, energy level, stress, and cortisol. Research indicates a few minutes per week in zone 5 can have health benefits. However, I have a client with mold exposure and high stress levels. She is not performing HIIT until the mold issue has been addressed with her practitioner. Instead, I have her walking and strength training two to three days per week. This demonstrates the importance of bio-individuality. High intensity can be useful for fat burning without sacrificing muscle and for situations where you need to exert yourself such as sprinting upstairs when the elevator is broken to make an appointment. However, the individual needs are always considered first.

A Sample Training Plan for Midlife Women

Here is an example of a full body workout done with dumbbells and bodyweight that is great for a woman in midlife.

Do each exercise without stopping. Rest 60 seconds, and repeat two more times to make three total sets or rounds

- Dumbbell chest press—15 reps
- Dumbbell overhead push press—15 reps
- Dumbbell rows—15 reps
- Tricep bench dips—20 reps
- Dumbbell front squat—15 reps
- Dumbbell walking lunges—30 steps
- Dumbbell bench step-ups—12 reps per leg
- Rest 60 seconds and repeat two more times for three total sets

A Word About Exercise Frequency as We Age

What about the later decades of life? Most of this book pertains to perimenopause and the transition into menopause. Do we need to continually change our training style and frequency as we move into a new decade of life?

Most of the principles concerning exercise intensity, frequency, and recovery can be followed as we advance in age. There may be some needed adjustments to frequency and how much time we spend with lifting, cardio, and movement. Movement constitutes activities that are not necessarily cardio in nature and tend to be lower impact. Having daily movement is beneficial at any age or stage of life.

There were two studies that looked at the best exercise frequency for women 60-plus years old when it comes to both strength training and cardio. Both studies compared groups who worked out one, two, and three times per week. The one-time-per-week group did one strength training and one cardio session. The two-times-per-week did two cardio and two strength training sessions. The three-times-per-week per week group did three strength training and three cardio sessions per week.

The first study found no difference in strength benefits between the three groups per week. The second study found a significant difference in energy expenditure with doing two training sessions per week (two strength training and two cardio sessions). The bottom line is there are no consistent results with these studies. However, we can surmise that there was no loss in strength between two weekly workouts as opposed to three weekly workouts.

Energy expenditure is higher in a 24-hour period when we are active throughout the day and not just during designated workout times.

Rest and Recovery

An important aspect of muscle growth, retention, and repair is rest and recovery. Muscle development occurs during times of rest and not when we are actively working the muscles. Whenever you lift in a way that stimulates and challenges the muscles, it forces an adaptation on the part of your body. The muscles must adapt and change to accommodate the new demands. Your muscles increase when the right amount of stress is placed upon them. This is why it's important to lift heavy enough and use other techniques such as supersets and burn-out sets to progressively overload the muscles. Progressive overload is simply a practice of gradually increasing the amount of tension and stress on muscles in order to force an adaptation that results in muscle growth.

However, in order to progress, attention to recovery is just as important as the training itself. As mentioned, muscles do not grow during the workout. They develop as we rest. When we lift, we make small microtears in the muscle that are repaired during the recovery phase. The repair results in an adaptation and greater muscle gains.

When a woman reaches perimenopause, this principle still applies. However, proper recovery becomes even more important than it was in her twenties and thirties. With age, our bodies do not recover as quickly. When you add hormonal changes to this, recovery becomes even more crucial. Women begin to experience problems regulating the hormone cortisol in their forties. This stress hormone can become too high or too low. It can also be high when it's supposed to be low (in the evening) and low when it should be high (in the morning). In general, women in perimenopause do not adjust to physical or emotional stress as quickly.

Exercise is an amazing tool for longevity and quality of life. However, like any tool, you will not reap the full benefits if you use it incorrectly. There are studies which have indicated that women over 50 do better with 72 hours rest between strength training sessions. For this reason, full body workouts can be helpful. However, this principle does not apply to every woman. Once again, bio-individuality is a consideration. Some women recover more quickly than others. However, there are a few principles to prevent over-training.

- Soreness—if your level of soreness after a workout is extremely high and lasts for days, this is an indication that either the training was too stressful or more recovery is needed. On a scale of 1 to 10 with 10 being extremely sore and 1 being not at all, I aim to be at a level 3 in soreness.

- Disruptions in sleep—this typically happens with long endurance cardio performed late in the day. Cortisol is released in the evening causing difficulty falling and staying asleep.
- Extreme fatigue—it's normal to be somewhat tired after a workout. However, if you are completely wiped out and don't want to leave the couch, you probably have over-trained.
- Allow 48 to 72 hours before training the same muscle group. You will want to pay attention to how long it takes your muscles to recover after a lifting session. If you are too sore or fatigued, you are actually depleting muscle gains rather than facilitating them. Glutes can be trained more frequently. These muscles tend to respond well to a higher volume of reps, sets, and frequency. Abdominals are considered endurance muscle fiber. They too can have a higher frequency of training.
- Cardio has a place, but too much endurance-based activity will release excess cortisol. Your body doesn't know whether it's out for a run or fleeing a cougar. It responds the same. Lots of zone 2 cardio is fine but watch that your heart rate is not elevated too high for too long. A general measure of maximum heart rate is 220 minus your age. Zone 2 is about 64 percent to 75 percent of that number. I am 61, so my maximum heart rate is 159 and my zone 2 is about 102 to 119 beats per minute. However, note that everyone is different.

Keep lifting sessions under an hour, not including warm up or time spent chatting with a friend at the gym. If you turn your resistance training into an endurance workout, you will not see the muscle growth.

You may be asking what exactly constitutes rest and recovery. Quality sleep is the main pillar for recovery. As mentioned in the intermittent fasting chapter, cellular repair occurs while we are at complete rest and not consuming food. On days you are not lifting or doing HIIT cardio, I suggest both active and passive recovery. Active recovery includes walking, restorative yoga, and foam rolling. Passive recovery includes massage, sauna, and the jacuzzi. I believe that daily exercise or movement is essential for health. However, not every day should include high intensity training or long endurance sessions.

Something I have frequently seen in my perimenopausal clients is adrenal dysfunction. Women in their forties are typically working, raising a family, and caring for aging parents. The demands of life combined with over-exercising and cortisol dysregulation can lead to adrenal dysfunction. For this reason, I often recommend that clients have cortisol levels checked. The Dutch test is excellent for this because it gives the cortisol levels for various times of day.

More on Exercise and Adrenal Dysfunction

As a way to convince you to incorporate recovery between workouts, we also need to consider the risk of adrenal dysfunction in perimenopause and menopause. As you'll soon realize, recovery between workouts is critical when we're in our forties, fifties, and above.

You may have heard of adrenal fatigue. This term is not recognized by Western medicine. However, hypothalamic-pituitary-adrenal (HPA) axis dysfunction is recognized and refers to the same symptoms. HPA dysfunction occurs when you have been pushing yourself for weeks or months without a break. Long periods of high stress can result in low levels of cortisol. When you override fatigue with caffeine, over-exercise, undereating, continual poor sleep, and continual extreme levels of stress, the HPA axis system will break down.

The hypothalamic-pituitary-adrenal (HPA) axis is part of the endocrine system. The HPA axis acts as a chemical messenger in the body. It consists of the hypothalamus, the pituitary gland, and the adrenal glands. When you face stress, the HPA axis system creates a stress response that leads to the release of a hormone called corticotropin (CRH). CRH triggers the release of the adrenocorticotropic hormone (ACTH) from the pituitary gland. ACTH then travels through the bloodstream down to the adrenal glands, where it triggers the release of the steroid hormone cortisol. Cortisol prepares the body for any potential threats by releasing a surge of glucose (blood sugar) for energy and suppressing the hormone insulin.

Think of the HPA axis as a feedback loop. When the hypothalamus and pituitary gland receive signals that high levels of cortisol have been released, they stop production of CRH and ACTH. This ceases the production of cortisol from the adrenals and stops the stress response. At this point, the body calms down, and hormone levels return to normal.

When the body is under constant, chronic stress, dys-function can occur in this feedback loop. Hormones continue to be released and can cause the glands of the HPA axis to become desensitized. As a result, the glands do not recognize or respond to the signal that would cease the production of hormones. Over time, this can lead to the condition known as "adrenal fatigue" or HPA axis dysregulation.

When the adrenal glands are not productive, this causes symptoms to occur during periods of prolonged stress or during (or after) acute or chronic infections. The term "adrenal fatigue" is not entirely accurate because the adrenal glands are only part of the problem. In reality, the entire HPA axis is malfunctioning. Thus, the whole feedback loop must be treated in order to relieve the symptoms.

The symptoms of HPA axis dysfunction can include:

- Sleep problems and insomnia
- Difficulty waking up in the morning
- Thyroid issues
- Inflammation
- Low immune system
- Blood sugar dysregulation
- Increase in abdominal fat
- Brain fog
- Extreme fatigue that is not relieved with quality sleep
- Dry skin
- Low libido
- Poor muscle tone
- Depression and anxiety
- Cravings for salty food
- Fatigue

Cortisol and DHEA are two of the adrenal hormones that have genetic influences on the body. They penetrate the cells to enter the nucleus, where DNA is unlocked. Cortisol is critical for health because it is the main hormone that directs immune function. Both DHEA and cortisol are involved in carbohydrate, protein, and fat metabolism, regulation of the immune system, hormone balance, and bone and neural tissue health.

The balance of cortisol levels in the body is important. Both high and low cortisol levels can cause health problems at the cellular level. The combination of elevated levels of cortisol and low levels of DHEA results in a chronic stress response. The body loses the ability to regulate essential functions, which can lead to hormone, immune, and metabolic breakdown. This has several effects on the body, including disrupted sleep, memory and cognitive problems, excess body fat, increased risk of infection, autoimmune disease from inflammation, and accelerated aging.

There are three stages to HPA axis dysfunction:

1. Cortisol increases and DHEA decreases. The balance between testosterone and estrogen is disrupted.
2. High levels of ACTH lead to a further decrease in DHEA and an eventual decrease in cortisol.
3. Cortisol and DHEA continue to decrease while high levels of ACTH remain. The adrenal glands have become exhausted and lose their ability to produce cortisol. This can cause the HPA axis to breakdown.

Rather than guessing (or attempting to self-diagnose) whether you have or are on the road to having HPA axis dysfunction, I suggest working with your medical provider or functional medicine doctor to test adrenal activity using saliva and dried urine. From there, your doctor may use herbal support, adaptogens, nutrients, and amino acids. In addition, it's important to address the stress, which initially caused the dysregulation.

Exercise may require a different approach when dealing with adrenal dysfunction. I recommend that clients do restorative yoga, walking, and low-level strength training sessions of 30 minutes or less. I also encourage them to do any resistance training earlier rather than later in the day.

High intensity interval training should be avoided until the dysregulation is addressed.

Exercise is critical to our health as we navigate through perimenopause into menopause. Muscle loss occurs when we lose estrogen, testosterone, and growth hormone. If we are not proactive, this muscle loss can lead to insulin resistance, excess adipose (body fat) tissue, loss of strength, and deterioration of bone density. Strength training is the best way to strengthen bones, increase skeletal muscle, and decrease the likelihood of metabolic disease from obesity. It should be a non-negotiable for every woman over the age of 40.

We have discussed how to navigate the physical stress of exercise in a way that creates a healthy, strong body. What about other types of stress? Perimenopausal women are more vulnerable to all types of stress, both physical and emotional. In the next chapter, we will dive into how midlife women often come face to face with unresolved past trauma and how hormonal shifts can contribute to this.

Chapter 6

The Story of Unresolved Trauma and Menopause

When I first began coaching women in health and fitness, I was focused more on aesthetics. How could I help them become the most physically fit, youthful-looking version of themselves at any age? While this is still a priority, I've learned that there are obstacles to a woman's health that go beyond what's on the end of her fork or how many times she can make it to the gym in a given week.

Debbie reached out to me for coaching a little over two years ago. Debbie was an intelligent woman who held a position in a prestigious law practice. She was no stranger to lifting weights or to eating whole, unprocessed food. In fact, she had quite a bit of knowledge surrounding exercise and nutrition. Since turning 50, she had gradually begun to put on excess weight. At age 54, her goal was to lose 40 pounds and increase lean muscle mass.

I started with the obvious changes of balancing her macro count and developing a strength training program she could fit into her busy lifestyle. As the days turned into weeks, Debbie began to slowly lose weight. Rather than being happy about the weight loss, she shared with me that it frightened her. Debbie opened up to me about past trauma and her internal struggle with emotional eating.

Debbie had a history of domestic and sexual childhood abuse. Early in life she had developed a pattern of disordered eating and excessive exercise to control her weight. In her early forties, she was viciously attacked and raped. She tried to bury the trauma, and at age 50 felt she had left the abuse in the past. However, it reemerged in the form of dreams, flashbacks, and unwelcome negative thoughts. The pounds began to creep on to her small frame. Debbie admitted to me that gaining weight had become a way to deter men from looking at her. The extra pounds felt safe, and as she lost weight, it conjured up feelings of insecurity and shame.

I knew from my own past experience with trauma that Debbie needed more than macros and dumbbells. I encouraged her to seek professional counseling. Over the course of a year Debbie worked with me on developing healthy eating and exercise habits. Her counselor helped her process and cope with past trauma. She lost an average of one pound per week while putting on a significant amount of skeletal muscle. The shape of her body completely changed. She gained confidence and swapped her baggy clothes for stylish, attractive outfits. She began highlighting her hair and wearing makeup. Debbie was no longer afraid to be beautiful, fit, and strong.

There is something that happens to women as they transition into menopause. Disappointment, pain, and unresolved trauma boil to the surface and cannot be ignored. They become more vulnerable to the effects of stress and dysregulation of cortisol levels. I've seen this in myself and in some of the women I've coached over the years.

There is even research to indicate that menopausal symptoms are heightened in women with past trauma. These women are three times more likely to have difficulty sleeping and twice as likely to experience decreased libido. There is a theory that menopausal symptoms in and of themselves are a trigger for women with past trauma. For example, experiencing hot flashes could potentially cause a sense of losing control, reminiscent of what was experienced in past trauma. As a woman who has gone through both trauma and extreme menopausal symptoms, I can say this was true for me.

There is a point of readiness as far as processing trauma. Dr. Aimie Apigan is a leading medical expert on how life experiences are stored in the body. She asserts that trauma becomes a part of our biology and that we must learn to practice regulation and connecting to our bodies first before processing the long-term effects of trauma on the nervous system.

Transitioning to menopause is often a time when the kids are moving from high school into college or careers. The empty nest is upon us. With a drop in estrogen, we lose our physiological propensity for "people pleasing." It's also a time when the physical symptoms of menopause may trigger past memories. I believe that all these factors converge and make processing trauma a must. The avoidance mechanisms of the past no longer work. For me, it was as if my body was screaming at me and saying, "Now is the time! You can no longer avoid me!" All the marathons, boot camps, and bodybuilding competitions in the world could not heal this inner brokenness.

Sometimes I wonder if my mother ever felt the weight of disappointment and unresolved trauma in her body. I think she did. There were days she shared with me desires and aspirations I never knew existed. She would often say to me, "Someday I will travel to London," or "Someday I'm writing a book." Someday never came for her.

My entire life I have struggled with anxiety. Instead of seeking help, I tried to hide it. I was ashamed of my anxiety and did everything I could to mask it. I saw it as a defect, a flaw, and a sign of weakness. I would avoid situations that intensified my feelings of anxiety. I buried childhood experiences, which had molded me into the defensive, frightened woman that I had become.

In my thirties and forties, I lapsed into a pattern of over-exercising to deal with the pain. The longer I cycled, ran, and hiked, the more I felt numb and exhausted. I was too exhausted for feelings, and that was precisely what I wanted.

I would like to tell you that my physical transformation from skinny runner to national bodybuilder was the point when I had my mental transformation. It simply isn't true. It would take me another four years to hit rock bottom emotionally and realize I couldn't outrun the past. There were marital problems, extreme anxiety, and depression. I made poor decisions and felt as if I was suddenly losing control of my life. It seemed as if everything had come full circle, and I was once again the scared little girl in the room with no windows. This was when I sought help.

At age 54, I was diagnosed with post-traumatic stress disorder. There was no more running or spending hours in the gym to hide. I needed a life raft, and this was exactly what my therapist gave me. I clearly remember the day she gave her diagnosis. I argued with her. I had parents who loved me. The things that happened in my childhood weren't "that bad." The abuse I suffered from a narcissistic man was not as horrible as what other women go through. In my mind, I felt I deserved nothing better, and to call my past "traumatic" was an exaggeration. I would be two years into therapy before I realized the truth.

As I write this book almost seven years later, my marriage is stronger than ever. I still struggle with anxiety and flashbacks. But the flashbacks are fewer and further between, and I now have the tools to manage my anxiety.

The stress I experienced took a physical toll on my body. For the first time in my life, I had cystic acne, a painful inflammatory acne condition causing pimples to form deep under the skin. How this condition happens is that the stress hormone cortisol is stimulated by a hormone in the brain called CRH. CRH binds to oil glands in the skin, causing excess oil production which blocks pores and produces inflammation. During those two years, I also suffered from hypothyroidism (most likely Hashimoto's) and rheumatoid arthritis flareups. I had continual urinary tract infections and was forced to be on antibiotics for almost a year.

I don't need research studies or science to tell me what stress can do to a woman's body in menopause. I lived it.

Today I am a big proponent of stress management and therapy. We live in a society where stress is not only normalized, it's seen as a mark of a successful person. Throughout my years of despair, I continued to train hard and compete. I continued to work with clients. I forged forward, but I was broken.

Stress can keep us in fight or flight with our sympathetic nervous system continually aroused. This causes cortisol to rise, which can result in weight gain, higher blood glucose, dysregulated insulin, and a lower immune system. As women, we need to honor where we are in time and space. Exercise is an amazing tool for health and potential longevity. Intermittent fasting has incredible cellular health benefits as well as possibly preventing chronic disease. However, if we are under extreme stress, we may need to adjust our exercise mode and frequency. We may also need to forgo fasting for a season. Managing stress first is non-negotiable.

In the rest of this chapter, we'll look at the biological mechanism of stress.

The Adrenals

Our brain has several areas that influence our emotional and psychological health. This includes the hypothalamus and the pituitary gland. The two work in conjunction to instruct glands in the body and influence our nervous system, emotional responses, immune system, and endocrine system.

The hypothalamus is the part of the brain that links the endocrine and nervous systems together. The pituitary gland controls both and is called the master gland. It receives signals from the hypothalamus and produces hormones, which act on the endocrine glands.

The adrenal glands are about the size of a walnut and sit on top of the kidneys where they secrete hormones such as cortisol and epinephrine. The adrenals are responsible for our stress response in the body, immunity, blood sugar regulation, fat storage and mobilization for energy and metabolism, and libido, and they are the hormones in charge of reproduction.

The three main hormone groups the adrenals are responsible for are mineralocorticoids (aldosterone), glucocorticoids (cortisol), and androgens (DHEA and testosterone) with cortisol being the most known. As described in chapter 1, cortisol performs many necessary functions such as helping with immune function, aiding in memory, and increasing blood sugar.

Cortisol gets a bad reputation. When it hangs out with insulin, these two hormones are often referred to as the "hormone bullies." The reality is that cortisol is critical. One of its main functions is associated with our stress and survival response.

Problems occur when cortisol is out of balance. For example, if it's chronically high in the evening and low in the morning, then this can cause sleep disturbances, digestive issues, cravings, brain fog, wrinkles, metabolic syndrome, and low thyroid function.

Adrenal issues are often related to our response to stress and perceived stress. Stress is regulated by a group of hormones and neurotransmitters that connect our brain and our body. In our current society, most of us are not balanced between the sympathetic (fight or flight) nervous system and the parasympathetic (rest and digest) nervous system. When we are in a sympathetic state, we experience anxiety, a sense of threat, anger, hypervigilance, restlessness, and insomnia. If we are in the parasympathetic state, we feel secure, calm, present, grounded, and connected.

Many women are dwelling in the sympathetic state and continually reacting with a fight-or-flight response even when danger is not imminent. This depletes the body of magnesium and selenium, which are responsible for thyroid function. Inflammation increases and our ability to create active from inactive thyroid hormone is diminished. We also will have a problem with the detoxification of estrogen from our bodies. When in chronic stress, our guts can become increasingly more permeable, and we can become vulnerable to food sensitivities.

There is also a third state referred to as the dorsal vagal freeze. It is also a survival mechanism, but it's a low energy state. This is where a person goes into a "freeze" state and feels exhausted, depressed, and overwhelmed. This state occurs when the threat seems too big or goes on too long.

We have to learn to manage these three states and to bring ourselves back to the middle parasympathetic area and maintain this state.

When in the "freeze" state, the body shuts down, and there is a disassociation from the body. The effects of the trauma remain in the nervous system. The effects can remain in the body and cause anxiety, depression, chronic fatigue, and chronic pain. Because the nervous system is in a state of dysregulation, every system controlled by the nervous system experiences the effects of the trauma. Biological effects of trauma can manifest as restlessness, immune system issues, inflammation, heart rate variability, metabolism, sleep disturbances, digestive problems, insulin resistance, depression, anxiety, and poor memory. These can potentially progress to medical diseases such as autoimmune and cardiovascular disorders.

According to statistics, 75 percent of Americans have moderate to severe stress. Over 40 percent of US adults suffer from health problems caused by stress. Women are more impacted by the effects of stress than men, and the impact is greater in perimenopause because of the dysregulation of cortisol and fluctuations in progesterone levels. Prior to perimenopause, our bodies are better at buffering stress because we have optimal levels of progesterone. Women in perimenopause experience months where ovulation does not occur. As a result, progesterone is low, causing increased anxiety and a decrease in quality sleep. In addition, decreased estrogen levels cause increased cortisol secretion. When estrogen and progesterone levels are low, the adrenal glands work hard to produce small amounts of progesterone and the precursors of estrogen. Ongoing stress combined with the strain on the adrenal glands can lead to adrenal dysfunction. It's important to recognize the signs of unresolved trauma since this can cause additional physical and mental stress on a woman's body.

Post-Traumatic Stress Disorder (PTSD)

Post-traumatic stress disorder can affect anyone at any point in life. However, there is a specific way that PTSD collides with the hormonal changes associated with perimenopause and menopause. A 2017 study published in *The Journal of Clinical Psychiatry* found that women who experience at least two adverse childhood events are twice as likely to experience depression in perimenopause, even if they had previously never had depression. Childhood adverse events in this study included divorce, marital separation, emotional or physical abuse, neglect, and substance abuse.

The Journal of the Menopause Society published research findings, which indicated menopausal symptoms are worsened by a past history of physical abuse. The study followed 682 women over the course of two decades from the child bearing years to menopause. The women who had experienced physical abuse decades earlier showed signs of anxiety and depression in menopause. The reason why midlife women who experienced past trauma have greater physical hormonal symptoms and mood disorders is unclear. However, one theory is that past traumatic experiences affect neurological health by affecting the brain, and the brain is a major part of hormonal production and signaling.

Post-traumatic stress disorder (PTSD) is caused by physical, sexual, and emotional abuse as well as military combat and life-threatening situations. People with PTSD recall traumatic events long past the event with flashbacks, nightmares, and intense thoughts. They often avoid people and places associated with the trauma. They can be hypervigilant and experience depression, anxiety, and anger. It can be as if the past is existing within the present.

Losing that sense of safety causes the fight-or-flight response to not only ramp up but to get stuck. The fight-or-flight alerts continue long after the danger has passed. According to Dr. Daniel Amen, the traumas become "branded in the brain." Brain single-photon emission computed tomography (SPECT) imaging studies have revealed that people who have PTSD tend to have too much activity in these areas of the brain:

- Deep limbic area—the brain's emotional center
- Basal ganglia—the brain's anxiety center
- Anterior cingulate gyrus—the brain's gear shifter (Imagine getting stuck on certain thoughts and behaviors.)

After being diagnosed with PTSD, one of the best skills my therapist taught me was how to move my responses from the amygdala to the prefrontal cortex. The amygdala is an almond-shaped mass of gray matter inside each cerebral hemisphere. The amygdala is believed to be the core of a neural system for detecting threats and processing fear. The amygdala also processes emotions such as anger and pleasure. The prefrontal cortex is responsible for reasoning, problem solving, comprehension, impulse control, and creativity. The amygdala automatically activates the fight-or-flight response and signals our brain to produce stress hormones. In contrast, the prefrontal cortex regulates and controls our emotional responses to stress and can help us to see stressful events as a little less of a threat.

I have found that awareness is key to moving my response to a situation from the amygdala to the prefrontal cortex in order to break the entrenched pattern of fear and hypervigilance. The three tools which have made the most difference for me are these:

- Changing my self-talk and inner dialog
- Prayer and meditation
- Journaling

Reframing our inner dialog is one of the best techniques for dealing with painful memories and flashbacks. For example, if I drive past a restaurant, which reminds me of an unpleasant event, I have an opportunity to change my thought process before those feelings overcome me. I can use my prefrontal cortex to logically categorize the situation by saying things like, "It's just a restaurant like any other restaurant. Good food is served there. Families and friends gather within those walls to celebrate birthdays and anniversaries. It's a place of laughter, not of sorrow." In this way, I help myself stay in my rational, logical mind instead of slipping down into the fear-focused amygdala.

Prayer and meditation are also powerful ways to bring awareness and find peace in the moment. When I have a conversation with God, it takes away the power of a disturbing thought or memory. It's hard to feel fear, anxiety, or shame when I am thanking God and asking for His protection.

Journaling was my least favorite way of dealing with trauma. However, at the insistence of my therapist, I agreed to try. Ultimately, I've found it to be one of the most powerful techniques I've experienced for dealing with past trauma. It gives you absolute clarity. You are able to see patterns. If you're carrying shame, the realistic depiction in your notes brings perspective and prevents you from shouldering that shame.

Before diving into any of these coping mechanisms, it's important to seek a licensed, professional therapist, who can help you navigate through the process. Digging up past trauma is painful. It's work. Evoking those emotions without someone to guide you can potentially cause you to relive painful or frightening experiences.

Last winter, I was at a live business event for online health coaches. One of the attendees told me about a business coach she had hired the previous year. She ended up leaving the program midway because of what she described as unethical practices. The coach was encouraging her students to dig into their clients' past traumas though they weren't at all trained in helping the clients process those traumas. It's important to note that this coach had absolutely no training in psychology, counseling, or trauma. She even played back one of her live coaching sessions with nutrition clients to demonstrate her point. In the call, women were breaking down into tears from the pain with no clear resolution on how to manage their trauma. The wounds were opened without any inkling of how to administer first aid.

As a health and fitness coach, I have encountered times that past trauma emerged in group discussions. This isn't surprising considering the connection between our mental and physical health. For example, it's believed that depression and anxiety affect the balance of the gut microbiome. When strong painful emotions emerged from my clients, my response was always to show empathy but encourage the woman to seek professional help. This is why I speak so openly about my experience with therapy. I want to remove the stigma of mental health and allow women to realize there is no shame in seeking counseling.

Generational Trauma

While generational trauma is not something specific to midlife women, it's important to touch on its potential impact. Our parents' anxieties and fears are often passed down through certain behaviors and genes. Just as physical characteristics are passed down, research has shown that traumatic experiences can also be passed down. Children of a parent struggling with PTSD are three times more likely to have PTSD themselves. Generational trauma can be present in families where divorce, abandonment, tragedy, substance abuse, suicide, abuse, and neglect have occurred.

Remember the woman I described at the beginning of this book in the preface? She was raised by two parents who suffered extreme trauma. That trauma was lived out over and over again in that old, moldy house. Her father's survival guilt and her mother's lifetime of suppressed anger and disappointment became part of a pattern, which would be passed down to the next generation. Ancestral and generational trauma can be stopped, but the trauma must be addressed.

The effect of generational trauma was first discovered with the adult children of Holocaust survivors who were seeking help with psychiatric problems associated with the hypervigilance and heightened response system you would see in PTSD. Originally this was believed to be because of the parents themselves. The parents were experiencing the effects of post-traumatic stress disorder, and the children were witnessing their parents' behavior in much the same way I did as a child. However, some research began to indicate that epigenetic changes could be transmitted to the children through the sperm, causing a heightened stress response. There was a possibility that trauma could leave a chemical mark on an individual's genes, which was passed down to subsequent generations. It doesn't damage the gene. Rather, it alters the mechanism by which the gene is expressed (epigenetics). The psychiatric problems can extend for up to three generations. Research is in its infancy, and nothing is conclusive. However, most of us can agree that being raised by a parent who experienced trauma may impact a child's perceptions and reactions in their developing years.

What does this mean to a midlife woman, and why is it important for her to consider generational trauma? Many midlife women are raising children at the same time they are dealing with their own stressors such as hormonal shifts, aging parents, and career demands. When life is busy and stress is high, it is easy to fall into dysfunctional patterns from childhood. If those patterns are rooted in her past trauma, they can be unconsciously passed down to her children. If the theory of epigenetic changes holds true, her children could experience many of the same symptoms of trauma. It's important to recognize these familial patterns of trauma and to have open and caring communication between generations. My parents grew up in a time when such things were never discussed or acknowledged. In writing this book, my hope is that there will be families who will have awareness and the loving conversations necessary to break the pattern of trauma.

We all carry within us a certain amount of past trauma. It doesn't always need to be classified as a large trauma such as a car accident, combat situation, or rape. There are mini traumas referred to as small "T" traumas, such as parental divorce or infidelity, which affect our mental wellbeing and keep us stuck in the fight-or-flight mode. Much of what constitutes trauma is perception. Because of increased cortisol and the loss of progesterone (our calming hormone), midlife women become vulnerable to the stress of past trauma. Through awareness and coping mechanisms, we can move into the more peaceful parasympathetic state in our body.

When I first began coaching midlife women on exercise and nutrition, past trauma was the furthest thing from my mind. Then I began to see numerous women with either adverse childhood experiences or a history of sexual and physical abuse. Often, they had not even shared this past trauma with their partner. For example, studies indicate that obese women aged 35 to 64 are more likely to have experienced past sexual abuse. In addition, research has shown that sleep disruptions are more severe in women who have a history of PTSD. When the effects of past trauma are combined with hormonal changes in perimenopause, sleep can suffer. Sleep is critical for cellular and brain health. In the next chapter, I discuss the effects of hormonal changes on sleep.

Chapter 7

Sleep

When I first met Jill, she was 47 years old and experiencing perimenopausal symptoms such as weight gain, moodiness, anxiety, and poor sleep. She was only sleeping an average of 5 hours per night. Even when she could fall asleep, she was waking frequently at night. During the day she was busy with a demanding job in the medical field and keeping track of her two preteen sons. She had put on 15 pounds over the past two years and was continually exhausted. Because her energy was low, she was using caffeine to get through her days. She found herself craving highly refined carbohydrates and sugary sweets. In an attempt to control her weight, she was doing excessive amounts of endurance cardio in the form of running and cycling for hours at a time, yet the number on the scale simply would not budge.

Over the course of 12 weeks, Jill and I worked on balancing her macros and eliminating snacking. She implemented sleep hygiene habits such as dimming artificial light after 6:00 p.m. in the winter months, putting away electronics at least one hour before bed, and establishing a nighttime routine, which included hot baths and a few minutes of meditation. Jill also made sure that her last meal was three to four hours prior to bedtime to allow time for digestive rest and glucose reduction. At the conclusion of 12 weeks, Jill lost 13 pounds and a significant amount of body fat in the midsection. More importantly, she was sleeping seven to eight hours most nights. Eliminating the nighttime snacking and putting away electronic devices were the two things, which made the greatest impact.

There is a stigma surrounding sleep. It is associated with laziness and lack of productivity. Lack of quality sleep has become a "badge of honor" and the norm for our modern-day society. According to Dr. Matthew Walker, we have lost 20 to 25 percent of our sleep over the past 70 years.

But the reality is that insomnia affects our physical and mental wellbeing. It has been associated with memory problems, mental health issues, and Alzheimer's risk. Guinness has banned setting the world record for sleep deprivation because of the associated dangers to physical and mental health.

To give some perspective, look at some of the other record breakers that are allowed by Guinness. For example, Felix Baumgartnerk went up in a hot air balloon to the outer surface of the Earth and then jumped out. He fell over 1,000 kilometers per hour and broke the sound barrier. This was NOT banned, yet Guinness banned sleep deprivation as being too dangerous. This should tell us something. Sleep is critical for health.

For me personally, I learned at an early age that sleep was something to be avoided. Sleep meant the ghosts walked the hallways and the monsters were under the bed. Sleep meant something bad might happen that was out of my control. When the little girl from this book's preface became a woman, sleep was still something she dreaded each and every night. Then when the young woman became the midlife woman, sleep became an impossibility as it was not only fraught with past trauma but also with biological issues at play from perimenopause and menopause.

In perimenopause it is common to experience sleep disturbances. Melatonin levels decrease sharply in women at age 40 and again at age 50. By the time we reach 60, we are barely producing melatonin. Melatonin is not a supplement. It is a complex hormone naturally released by the pineal gland in the brain. It helps to regulate your 24-hour sleep-wake cycle known as the circadian rhythm. Its release is triggered by darkness, causing the body temperature and respiration to lower in preparation for sleep. However, melatonin is involved in more than our sleep. It is also produced in the gut where it is believed to be associated with intestinal motility and the immune system. It is also thought to play a role in reproduction, sex hormones, the timing of menopause, and serotonin levels. Serotonin is a chemical involved in sleep, digestion, bone health, healing, and sexual desire. In addition, melatonin is believed to be a powerful antioxidant (a compound that can prevent cell damage) and is twice as active as vitamin E in preventing inflammation. Lower levels of melatonin in perimenopause and menopause are a cause of concern, especially when combined with higher cortisol.

As women we become more vulnerable to the effects of stress and can experience cortisol dysregulation. When cortisol rises, so do blood glucose levels. Cortisol inhibits the release of insulin, making it more difficult to regulate blood sugar. When cortisol is high, our brain and body receive the message that it's daytime. Cortisol levels should be highest in the morning and lowest at night. Unfortunately for midlife women, this is not the case in our modern world. A combination of late-night eating, bright artificial lights, electronic devices, and stress work to raise cortisol and lower melatonin, creating a wakening response. In addition, chronically poor sleep has been linked with blood sugar dysregulation and insulin resistance, which can lead to diseases such as type 2 diabetes and heart disease.

In menopause, numerous factors affect sleep, including hormonal changes, night sweats, hot flashes, and mental health issues. Depression and anxiety are common in menopause and can impact sleep. Yet lack of sleep can, in turn, impact mental health. According to Dr. Sara Gottfried, women in perimenopause and menopause who experience night sweats and hot flashes are more likely to develop anxiety, decreased memory, problems with concentration, pain, and fearfulness. All of these factors can affect sleep, and lack of quality sleep affects our ability to manage hunger, cravings, and stress levels.

Lack of sleep has been associated in several ways with weight loss resistance. According to a 2021 study presented by the Endocrine Society, a combination of low estrogen with sleep disturbances can decrease the amount of fat used for energy. Over time, this leads to fat storage, weight gain, and weight loss resistance. Sleep deprivation also affects the hunger hormones leptin and ghrelin. Leptin decreases while ghrelin increases. Leptin is responsible for satiety, and it is believed to decrease as we age. Ghrelin increases our hunger response. The result of leptin decreasing and ghrelin increasing is increased cravings. One study found that sleep-deprived individuals craved high-fat and sugary foods following a sleepless night. Cortisol tends to remain higher in individuals deprived of sleep, and chronically high levels are associated with visceral fat, especially in the midsection. In addition, lack of sleep affects our ability and desire to exercise. Thus, there is a combination of hormonal fluctuations, increased cravings, and decreased desire or ability to exercise.

It is believed that chronic lack of quality sleep can accelerate the aging process. A University of California team found that one night of partial sleep deprivation activated genes related to biological aging. After a night of partial sleep deprivation, participants' blood levels showed signs of deterioration in the cell's growth and division cycle. Another study in mice indicated that lack of sleep adversely changed melatonin metabolism and increased levels of cortisol, phenylamine, and aspartic acid, which suppress the release of neurotransmitters in the brain. Optimal neurotransmitter balance is essential for health. Neurotransmitters are the language spoken by our brain. An imbalance can cause the body to be over- or under-stimulated, resulting in problems with everything from heart rate and movement to mood. Without neurotransmitters our neurons are unable to communicate, and we would not be able to live.

There are vital processes occurring in the brain when we sleep seven to nine hours. Brain cells are repaired. Toxins are flushed away. Neuronal connections that protect against deterioration are activated. These functions keep our brain working at optimum levels and promote emotional wellbeing. As we move through our day, an accumulation of waste products build up in our cells. Inflammation (a precursor to disease) builds up in our body and brain. Electrons can become toxic, leading to oxidative stress. Oxidative stress can cause damage to cells, proteins, and DNA, which contribute to aging. Cells repair only when we are sleeping. If we aren't sleeping, the toxicity and inflammation remain present.

Insomnia is defined as difficulty falling asleep or staying asleep. Chronic insomnia occurs when a person cannot sleep more than six hours a night and experiences attention issues at least three days per week for more than three months or over the course of years. Being female puts you at higher risk of insomnia.

There are cognitive issues related to insomnia. Researchers believe that the different sleep stages play a critical role in brain health. Sleep deprivation is associated with a decrease in blood flow to the brain affecting memory, learning, attention, reaction times, and judgment. It's also linked to depression, anxiety, and other mental health conditions.

Research indicates that insomnia is one of the most common conditions that impacts the brain. Sleep deprivation is associated with a decrease in blood flow to the brain. Sleep is a time when the brain selects memories and discards non-essential information. This happens during REM and NREM sleep. One study in the *Journal of Sleep Research* indicated that lack of sleep may cause the incorporation of false information into your memories.

North of forty, a woman needs to consider certain lifestyle habits to ensure she has better sleeping potential. For example, I recommend you consider the following:

- Nutrition and balance of macros (protein, carbs, and fats)—proper nutrition can help to balance hormones and reduce sleep problems. Always start each meal with adequate quality protein. Aim for 30 grams. Include healthy fats and fiber for blood sugar balance. At bedtime, it can be beneficial for sleep to include some low glycemic carbs. According to Dr. Alan Christianson, having low glycemic carbohydrates can prevent cortisol from raising blood sugar, which interferes with sleep and potentially causes a blood sugar crash resulting in cravings.
- Cortisol response with exercise—it's best to exercise earlier in the day to avoid spiking cortisol levels close to bedtime.

- Nighttime snacking—this can raise blood glucose levels and cortisol, so avoid it.
- An adequate window of time from the last meal until bedtime. We are less insulin sensitive at night, meaning we are less able to deal with increased blood sugar levels. Eating before bed raises blood glucose levels at a time where we are least able to regulate those levels. High blood sugar levels are a signal to the body that it's not at rest.
- Digital detox—do a digital detox from electronics and wear blue blockers in the evening.
- A nighttime routine—develop a nighttime routine for relaxation; for example, a cool room, dim the lights, and hot bath.
- Supplementation—talk to your practitioner about using a slow-release melatonin to improve total sleep time and quality of sleep.
- Stress management—DHEA and cortisol are two hormones responsible for managing stress levels. Both are secreted by the adrenal glands. As women transition into menopause, the ovaries cease to function and the adrenal glands take on the job of producing estrogen. When a midlife woman does not get quality sleep, this adds stress on the adrenals. They can become burdened, leading to adrenal dysfunction.
- Progesterone—work with your functional medicine provider to see if this is a good option for you. In menopause progesterone drops, which negatively impacts sleep. Natural progesterone can improve sleep.

Melatonin

Melatonin is a hormone which is vastly misunderstood. Dr. Stephen Gundry refers to melatonin as the "bouncer at the bar" for the mitochondria. You will see why after you read this section.

As mentioned prior, melatonin is more than just a sleep hormone. It impacts us at the cellular level. Melatonin becomes critical when we experience stress. When we experience stress, an adaptation is necessary as a protection mechanism. When your body encounters stress, it attempts to deal with the new demands by adapting and becoming more resilient. Any adaptation requires additional energy to be produced. For example, if we lift heavy enough weight to produce small micro tears in the muscle, an adaptation to this stress occurs as a protection mechanism: the muscles adapt by growing bigger and stronger. This process requires energy.

Diseases are believed to start when there is a lack of adequate energy within the body, meaning the mitochondria in the cells cannot meet the energy demands resulting from the physical stress. The mitochondria are extremely sensitive to stress and will eventually stop producing energy if they become overwhelmed with excessive physical stress. If this occurs, the rest of the cell is left to produce energy as best it can. Unfortunately, this does not work well. Underlying the onset of disease is a lack of energy for providing an adaptation response. Our physical health depends on our body's ability to be resilient and adapt to stress. If we cannot produce enough energy to adapt, disease and illness can occur.

When stress exceeds the body's ability to adapt, you start to have inflammation. All stress has an inflammatory nature. Inflammation is a natural occurrence designed to help our body heal. If you cut yourself, you may experience some swelling, and eventually a scab forms. In this case, the inflammation is a short-term acute response. However, inflammation becomes a problem when it is ongoing, and the inflammation faucet will not stop flowing. Eventually, the body can start to see its own tissues, joints, and organs as threats because of this excess inflammation. This occurs with type 2 diabetes and cardiovascular and autoimmune diseases such as Hashimoto's thyroiditis and rheumatoid arthritis. At the root of chronic disease is inflammation. According to the World Health Organization (WHO), this is the number one cause of death in the world.

Mitochondria are responsible for 90 percent of energy production inside cells. They are like a factory workforce for cells. We cannot survive without mitochondria. They play a critical role in energy metabolism in tissues, including the liver and the skeletal muscle. Mitochondria are associated with hormone production (estrogen, progesterone, testosterone, and cortisol). For example, cortisol production begins and ends in the mitochondria. They are involved in the production and release of neurotransmitters. Mitochondria turn inflammation on and off, which is an important part of controlling the disease process. If mitochondria cannot function, the cell becomes injured or dies.

As mentioned above, mitochondria do not like chronic inflammation. When it becomes too much for the mitochondria, they simply "check out." The energy production is then taken out of the mitochondria and produced in the rest of the cell, which only gives 10 percent of the energy of what mitochondria would produce under normal (non-stressful) conditions. Imagine only having 10 percent of your immune response properly working. This is what happens when we don't have the energy produced by the mitochondria. If mitochondria are damaged or unable to produce energy, cells will die, leaving us vulnerable to illness and disease.

This is where melatonin becomes critical. The melatonin residing inside the mitochondria prevents the mitochondria from making that switch in energy production away from the mitochondria to the cell where it would lose 90 percent of its energy. Melatonin is the key to holding the balance of energy production in the mitochondria. As mentioned before, it's a strong antioxidant made in every cell of the body that can protect the body against disease by potentially preventing cell damage. In lab experiments, antioxidant molecules have been shown to counteract the damage from free radicals such as cigarette smoke. By the age of 40 all of us have compromised or damaged mitochondria, and most of us have less melatonin than what we produced in earlier decades. If you add any chronic illness such as autoimmune disease to this, you have an inefficient energy system trying to deal with the energy needs of your body. Given the global pandemic, this problem has increased.

Melatonin is an incredible hormone that promotes brain health, immunity, anti-inflammatory function, and sleep. Pineal melatonin regulates the sleep and wake cycle and is a relatively small amount of melatonin compared to the total amount produced by the body. The pineal gland produces and stores melatonin during the light hours, which will be released during sleep. This natural cycle allows us to move into the parasympathetic nervous system (a body state that is calm and restful) as we approach the nighttime hours. It's how we repair our bodies when we sleep, including the brain and the cardiovascular system. When we lose the regeneration and repair time due to insufficient sleep, our ability to adapt to stress decreases. This, in turn, leads to the potential loss of energy produced by the mitochondria. It is melatonin that potentially gives us resilience and the ability to adapt to stress.

Electronic and magnetic fields (EMF) from our electronic devices and artificial light at night can interfere with this natural, innate process of sleep, which is part of our 24-hour circadian rhythm. Things such as blue-blocking glasses and sleep masks can help. However, in the later years of life, melatonin production declines regardless of these measures. Some doctors advocate for supplementation as we age, especially past age 60 when melatonin is virtually non-existent. However, if supplementing melatonin, it's important to choose a high-quality, trusted brand as opposed to one off the store shelf. Everyone responds differently to melatonin. It's advised to consult your healthcare provider.

Deep sleep is the primary activator of the lymphatic system. The lymphatic system helps our body to get rid of waste, and this is critical for our health and immunity. Not having enough deep sleep has been associated with the development of neuroinflammation (inflammation in the brain), cognitive decline, and mood disorders such as anxiety and depression. Research has shown that microglial cells have excessive activity without quality sleep. This activity can make the brain more vulnerable to damage. Sustained microglial cell activity has been observed in patients with Alzheimer's disease. Abnormal protein accumulation is one thing that neurologic conditions can have in common. The proteins are often a response of the immune system. For example, neurologic infections will produce these proteins (including Lyme disease and toxins). A government study found a correlation between chronic lack of deep sleep and these abnormal protein deposits.

Recently, it has been reported that melatonin can modulate specific gut microbiota activity. It has been shown that melatonin can influence the swarming and motility of human intestinal bacteria. The brain and the gut are connected by millions of nerves, in particular the vagus nerve. The vagus nerve provides a link between the central nervous system and the enteric nervous system, which is the largest part of the autonomic nervous system and orchestrates gastrointestinal behavior. A paper published by PubMed stated that the function of the bowel is so complex that it has its own intrinsic nervous system. Research is still in its infancy, and there is more unknown than known. However, because of the believed connection between the brain and the gut, it's important that we are mindful during times where we are under stress. This includes a focus on sleep and stress management.

Now, sleep is an absolute priority for me. I wear an Oura Smart Ring to track my sleep and am diligent about my bedtime. Gone are the night terrors I suffered with for most of my life. Gone is the sleepwalking (just like my dad). Gone are the night sweats from menopause. Yes, anxiety still comes calling when my head hits the pillow. Yes, the monsters sometimes peek out from under the bed, and the ghosts from that old, moldy house of my childhood try to enter the bedroom, but I've learned. I've learned how to quiet my mind and the fears that can keep me hypervigilant even to this day. I know sleep is essential for my longevity and health. How I survived five decades without it escapes me. I only know that if I can change my sleep patterns, so can you.

Sleep is a critical part of longevity and health span for both men and women. However, women face unique sleep challenges beginning in perimenopause and extending into menopause. It's one of the most common concerns I hear from the women I coach. At the very least, poor sleep causes weight gain and impaired memory. At its worst, the chronic stress of poor sleep can create cell damage, metabolic disease through insulin resistance, changes in the brain, a lower immune system, and even disease. In the next chapter we will be unpacking the role of supplements and how they can help with the challenges women encounter in perimenopause and menopause.

Chapter 8

Midlife Women and Supplements

Supplements can help to maximize your health and fitness results from proper nutrition, exercise, and sleep. However, it's important to understand the role of each supplement. Take my client, Iris, for example. She could never seem to reach her protein goals. She had a busy job in the finance department at a university. There were few breaks to eat because of her workload. Iris would often experience a midday lack of energy because she wasn't able to eat lunch. I encouraged her to include an afternoon smoothie made with a quality protein powder to help her meet her protein needs and prevent the fatigue she experienced. She added coconut milk, berries, and greens to her protein smoothie. I also suggested she add an additional scoop of protein to bring her closer to her protein goal and include a fiber powder supplement in her shake. The fiber would aid with satiation and fullness as well as blood glucose stability. After a week, she reported that the protein had helped to alleviate the hunger and fatigue in the afternoon. She was also finding it easier to meet her protein needs.

Supplementation taken correctly can help with sleep, energy, muscle synthesis, hydration, nutrition, and detoxification of the liver. Let's unpack a few of these supplements and how they can help you. Here are ones I have personally used and recommend to my clients.

Be sure to discuss these supplements with your healthcare provider, particularly if you are taking prescription medications. This information is for educational purposes only and does not constitute medical advice.

Electrolytes

Electrolytes are critical if you are following a low-carbohydrate eating plan or doing extended fasts. Electrolytes include minerals such as sodium, potassium, magnesium, and chloride, which affect every cell in your body. Fasting and lower carbohydrate eating plans can cause the loss of water and electrolytes in your body. This can, in turn, lead to headaches, body aches, and nausea.

Staying hydrated is critical because every cell in the body needs water and our daily metabolic processes use it. We are not able to store a supply of water in our body like we can when we consume food. Thirst declines with age, which increases the risk of dehydration. Dehydration causes a loss of elasticity in the skin, which contributes to sagging and wrinkles. When we transition to menopause, we lose estrogen. Estrogen helps to keep our skin supple. When it declines, we can experience dry and crepey skin. Electrolytes can help to hydrate the skin.

Many women find they do better with fewer carbohydrates after menopause. This is bio-individual. I have noticed that at age 61, my body does not assimilate carbs as well as it did even a decade ago. This is especially true in the case of blood sugar dysregulation and insulin resistance. For this reason, many women will opt to lower their carbohydrate intake when trying to lose body fat. We lose the electrolyte sodium through our urine when we are on a low-carb diet. Low sodium levels can increase cortisol levels, causing insomnia, weakness, and headaches. If you do not get enough sodium, you will also have problems absorbing magnesium, which is responsible for many vital body reactions. It's important to maintain the sodium-potassium water balance in the blood because it is how your body maintains fluid balance in the cells, extracellular fluid, and blood volume. For example, if sodium is too high and potassium is low, it can raise your blood pressure. It is rare in the US to see low sodium with high potassium, and it is mostly found in those with diabetes, chronic kidney disease, and cardiovascular disease.

Here are a few facts you may be surprised to learn about sodium:

- Sodium reduces hunger—salt cravings may actually mean you are low in sodium.
- Sodium aids in reducing insulin resistance—one of the key defense mechanisms in our body is to increase insulin levels in response to low sodium. It's believed that the body has an alarm or panic reaction when salt is too low. Insulin helps the kidneys to hold on to salt. Since insulin resistance is a condition affecting many midlife women, it's important to be aware of the things which increase glucose and insulin.

- Sodium improves digestion—the liver needs sodium to create bile salts, which assist the gut.
- Sodium boosts learning and concentration—your brain requires a normal salt balance to function. Lack of sodium slows the nervous system.
- Sodium gives you more energy.
- Sodium helps with bone health—one of the highest sodium sources in your body is your bones. Low sodium can cause the body to start dissolving bone in order to extract the sodium.

The electrolyte magnesium is responsible for over 300 bodily reactions; for example, maintaining normal nerve and muscle function, maintaining a healthy immune system, strengthening bones, regulating blood glucose levels, and regulating the heartbeat. Every organ in the body requires magnesium, especially the heart and the kidneys. According to research, as many as 10 out of 11 women are deficient in magnesium. A magnesium deficiency can damage our mitochondria. Since mitochondria are the working powerhouses of our cells, damage can lead to a low energy state, which causes us to become more susceptible to infection and chronic disease.

Magnesium is also important for the following:

- Reducing insulin resistance
- Curbing food cravings
- Increasing bone strength, which is important for women in perimenopause and menopause
- Maintaining brain health
- Maintaining cardiovascular health
- Regulating blood pressure

There are several forms of magnesium available in supplement form, and each can have different benefits. They include:

- Magnesium glycinate—it acts as an anti-inflammatory substance and can help with stress, anxiety, depression, insomnia, and constipation. This is my favorite form of magnesium because of the potential sleep and relaxation benefits.
- Magnesium malate—it is gentler and has less of a laxative effect than magnesium glycinate. It is used to treat fibromyalgia and chronic fatigue.
- Magnesium citrate—it has a natural laxative effect.
- Magnesium lactate—it absorbs in the gut easily and is gentler and well tolerated. It is used in individuals who need to supplement with a large amount of magnesium. It is also used to treat anxiety and stress.
- Magnesium chloride—it used to treat low magnesium, heartburn, and constipation.
- Magnesium taurate—it may help to promote healthy blood sugar levels and support healthy blood pressure.
- Magnesium L-threonate—it may support brain health, treat depression, and protect from memory loss.
- Magnesium orotate—it may promote heart health and energy production in the blood vessel tissue.
- Magnesium oxide—it used to treat digestive issues such as heartburn and constipation. However, it is poorly absorbed. Thus, this is not the best option for those who require greater amounts of magnesium.

- Magnesium sulfate (Epsom salt)—it dissolves in water and is used to treat stress and sore muscles.

Chloride is also an important electrolyte. It works with sodium and potassium to regulate and control fluids within the body. It impacts blood pressure and muscle function.

Years ago, I was preparing for a bodybuilding show. My carbohydrate intake was very low at the time. When I went to see my certified nurse practitioner for a checkup, I was stunned to find that my blood pressure was extremely low. Low blood pressure can cause dizziness, fainting, and even death. This is an example of an electrolyte imbalance in the body.

My favorite electrolyte supplement is LMNT (pronunciation is "element"), which dissolves easily in water. LMNT is an electrolyte powdered drink mix containing the perfect balance of sodium, potassium, and magnesium. Unlike many other electrolyte drinks, it's free of all sugar, gluten, and questionable additives. I should add that I am receiving no form of compensation for this recommendation or for any of the product recommendations I make in this book.

When you are fasting, use the unflavored electrolytes. Even stevia can break your fast. When you are in a feeding window, you can use the flavored choices.

Protein Powder

I believe we should obtain protein from real, whole, nutritious foods. However, I am also a realist. I know it can be difficult to get our protein requirements in during the day. This is particularly true with plant-based diets and with intermittent fasting. I prefer protein made from bone broth as opposed to whey. I experience bloating with whey, and many of my clients have reported the same.

As women age, we do not assimilate the amino acids from protein as well as we did in our twenties and thirties. As a result, we actually need to consume more protein to receive the benefit. This need continues to increase as we age. Once a woman transitions into menopause, she rapidly loses muscle and replaces it with adipose (body fat) tissue if she is not proactive with nutrition and strength training. I generally recommend that most women consume one gram of protein per pound of ideal body weight. This can be a challenging number to hit at times, especially if a woman is not accustomed to eating much protein. In my experience, most midlife women are not consuming enough protein, which is why I recommend supplementing with a high quality protein powder.

My two favorite protein powder supplements are the All-in-One Shake by JJ Virgin and Simply Protein: Bone Broth Protein by Cynthia Thurlow. I suggest 20 to 30 grams per serving. For example, with the JJ Virgin protein, two scoops equal 20 grams. In women struggling to meet their protein needs, I generally recommend three scoops to make 30 grams.

C60 Purple

C60 Purple is quickly becoming my favorite supplement for energy, clarity, and focus. C60 is short for carbon 60, a molecule made up of 60 tiny carbon atoms forming something that looks like a hollow soccer ball. Because it forms a spherical cage, it acts like a sponge, neutralizing harmful free radicals. Free radicals are unstable molecules that can cause damage to other molecules such as DNA. They have been linked to cancer. C60 is a recently discovered, Nobel Prize-winning molecule. C60 is found in nature and in the atmosphere of giant red stars. It is considered to be one of the most powerful antioxidants known. The company C60 Purple Power was founded by a biogeochemist and research scientist who has developed this product in both an oil and a gummy form.

C60 works at the cellular level to help the cells overcome oxidative stress. If you recall, oxidative stress occurs when there is an imbalance between free radicals that are damaging to the cells and antioxidants, which can fight free radicals. Causes of oxidative stress include toxins, pollutants, alcohol consumption, and obesity. C60 can help to optimize mitochondrial function. As mentioned throughout this book, the mitochondria are the powerhouses for energy production in the cells. As we age, the health of our mitochondria can decline. Fasting can help to increase cellular health through autophagy, which is the body's way of cleaning out damaged cells in order to regenerate new, healthy cells. In addition to fasting, C60 is a supplement that's valuable for potentially optimizing the mitochondria as well as helping us to maintain energy levels throughout the day.

According to the manufacturer of C60 Purple, it is safe to use with other medications and supplements. However, they do recommend consulting your doctor if you take a blood thinner to ensure the blood does not become too thin.

Fiber

Fluctuations in hormones during perimenopause can lead to glucose spikes and crashes, which can be a precursor to insulin resistance. Fiber reduces spikes and helps to stabilize blood sugar. In menopause, it is common for women to experience constipation as estrogen and estrogen receptors in the gastrointestinal tract decline, affecting the muscles in the colon. We don't always receive the amount of fiber our body needs from our diet. Thus, I recommend supplementing.

Fiber helps you to burn fat and maintain a healthy weight. It has protective qualities against type 2 diabetes, cardiovascular disease, and coronary heart disease. High fiber slows down stomach emptying and takes longer to move through the digestive tract. This will allow you to feel fuller on fewer calories than low-fiber foods. Fiber helps fat to move through the digestive system so that less is absorbed. Fiber also keeps blood sugar levels stable, which in turn allows for a steady amount of energy to the brain. One study looked at 345 overweight and obese adults who were on a calorie-restricted diet. Researchers found that higher fiber promoted weight loss and greater consistency with the diet independent of macronutrient and calorie counting.

Studies have also indicated that fiber promotes steady glucose (sugar) levels by preventing insulin spikes and crashes that are associated with type 2 diabetes. The risk of type 2 diabetes can be reduced by 20 to 30 percent according to this research. Fiber also stimulates insulin to suppress ghrelin, the hormone that tells you that you're hungry.

The trillions of bacteria that inhabit the gut thrive on fiber, and these bacteria have an effect on immune health and inflammation. Menopause alters the gut microbiome, which can lead to insulin resistance and a lower metabolism. Fiber can help reduce the bad kinds of bacteria by supporting the good bacteria in the gut. If gut bacteria are deprived of fiber, they will actually eat the intestinal lining as a source of food. This causes gut permeability and allows dangerous bacteria to penetrate the colon wall. Fiber can help maintain a thick mucus layer in the lining of the colon.

Fiber remains intact until it reaches the colon where it is fermented by bacteria and short-chain fatty acids (SCFAs) are produced. SCFAs are metabolic products that provide the energy source for the colon. They can also reduce damage from free radicals (such as toxins), lower inflammation, support immunity, and reduce the risk of cardiovascular disease. When women lose estrogen in menopause, they are at a greater risk of abnormal lipid levels and heart disease.

Dietary fiber is actually a carbohydrate, but your body does not convert it to sugar. The body does not have the digestive enzymes to break down fiber. It moves through the digestive system where some is fermented in the colon and others give the stools bulk.

There are three types of fiber. Soluble fiber absorbs water and can help maintain healthy cholesterol levels and stable blood sugar levels. Insoluble fiber remains whole and does not absorb water. It helps with healthy stools and quicker waste elimination. The third type is fermentable fiber, referred to as prebiotics. It supports healthy gut bacteria. Soluble fiber can also aid in detoxification of the digestive tract by killing off bad bacteria such as candida. Insoluble fiber can bind with carcinogens and other toxic chemicals that are formed when you digest food and eliminate waste through the feces.

Fiber can help lower inflammation. A major marker for inflammation is C-reactive protein (CRP). One study found that those with the highest fiber intake had a 63 percent lower risk of elevated CRP. Low-grade chronic inflammation begins in the gut and eventually becomes systemic. This type of ongoing inflammation is associated with almost every disease.

Recommended fiber is 25 to 30 grams per day. The average adult in the United States is only getting about 15 grams per day. Some statistics show that women are only consuming 12 grams per day. I recommend that my clients consume 50 grams per day. However, do not start with 50 grams per day. You need to give your digestive system a chance to adjust. Add five grams every other day until you reach 50 grams. Increase your water intake as well. You can get fiber from non-starchy vegetables, nuts, seeds, wild rice, beans, quinoa, and berries.

Because getting enough fiber from food alone is challenging, supplementing can help. Here are some of my favorite products: Simply Fiber by Cynthia Thurlow, Extra Fiber by JJ Virgin, and OptiFiber by Xymogen.

Activated B Complex

Activated B complex supports your body's methylation (detoxification) pathways and cellular health. Hundreds of bodily processes need vitamin B, and many of us are deficient in it. The methylation cycle is a biochemical pathway that performs many functions, including turning genes on and off, producing energy, reducing inflammation, immune function, and detoxification. Methylation is dependent on the B vitamins to help the liver and other organs convert and excrete toxins. About 40 percent of the population has a genetic anomaly that prevents the absorption of vitamin B. Activated simply means that each B vitamin is in its bioavailable form. Thus, supplementation can be helpful.

There are two phases of detoxification. In phase one, toxins are neutralized by enzymes and converted to a less harmful form. In order to protect the liver, in phase two they are converted to a safer water-soluble form for elimination from the body. It is important that toxins from processed food, your environment, and xenoestrogens (synthetic or natural chemical compounds that mimic estrogen) are in a safe form before they reach your gut for final elimination. A methylated or active form of B supports the pathways and helps the liver with this conversion process.

Active B complex is also important to help with potentially reversing estrogen dominance, which is common in perimenopause when hormone levels are fluctuating. Although estrogen may be low, the levels are high in relation to progesterone. These fluctuations can begin as early as 35 to 38 years of age when women will begin to skip an ovulation cycle. This leads to less progesterone because progesterone is produced during ovulation. Between the ages of 35 to 50 years, progesterone can decline by 70 percent. It can decline an additional 30 percent going into menopause. Signs of estrogen dominance include fibroids, ovarian cysts, weight gain, low libido, migraines, irregular periods, endometriosis, water retention, fatigue, heavy periods, and belly fat. Excess amounts of estrogen can be removed through the detoxification process. I purchase my activated B complex from Dr. Mariza Snyder.

Liver Support

As described above, the liver is responsible for detoxification from environmental toxins, excess estrogen, medications, and xenoestrogens. In menopause, reduction in estrogen combined with mitochondrial dysfunction associated with the aging process can create an environment that strains the liver. One paper by the *World Journal of Gastroenterology* described this as "an interplay of hormonal issues and aging that create a unique path for development of liver disease in menopausal women." A 2019 PubMed paper stated that estrogen deficiency has the potential to worsen non-alcoholic fatty liver disease (NAFLD) in mice models with fatty liver. While we are not mice, the study, combined with the prevalence of NAFLD in menopausal women, shows this is a valid concern for midlife women. It's important to show your liver lots of love. Here are my two absolutely favorite liver supplements:

Please note: The supplements suggested below are only available through a healthcare provider and cannot be purchased directly from the manufacturer. Thus, you will need to find a naturopathic or functional medicine practitioner who can prescribe them.

- Liver Protect—it helps with healthy immune function, antioxidant support, and detoxification.
- Advanced Tudca—of the two supplements, this is my "go to." I never run out. Tudca helps with detoxification, healthy digestion, drainage, and the support of bile production of the liver.

MCT Oil

MCT oil is a medium-chain triglyceride (MCT) that is different from other fatty acids. Fatty acids are the building blocks of the fats in our body. They are present in our bloodstream, the cells and tissues of our body, and in the dietary food that we eat. During digestion the body breaks down fats into fatty acids, which are then absorbed in the blood. Fatty acid molecules are usually joined in groups of three into a molecule called a triglyceride. Triglycerides are also made in the body from the carbohydrates we consume. Fatty acids perform many functions, including energy storage, modulation of gene expression, and responsiveness to hormonal signals. If glucose is not available, the body uses fatty acids as fuel for the cells.

Most of the fats we consume from animals and plants are long-chain triglycerides (LCT). They are found in meat, fish, avocados, seeds, and nuts. MCT oils are naturally occurring in goat milk, sheep milk, coconut oil, human breast milk, and palm oil. Because MCT oil is a medium chain fatty acid, it is more easily absorbed than LCTs. MCT oil does not require bile or pancreatic enzymes for digestion. It's transported to the liver for immediate energy. Long-chain fatty acids have to go through several steps to be digested and sent to the liver. Because MCT oil does not need to go through these steps and is more easily digested than LCTs. MCT oil can be beneficial for midlife women by providing a quick energy boost and the mental clarity that comes from this boost. As hormones fluctuate in perimenopause, women begin to have difficulty with brain fog. When a woman loses estrogen, she becomes more vulnerable to cognition problems, such as memory loss.

Fatty acids are classified based on the degree of saturation or unsaturation in the carbon chain. If there is no double bond, the fatty acid is saturated. If there is one double bond, the fatty acid is monounsaturated. If there are two or more double bonds, the fatty acid is polyunsaturated. Saturated fats can be short chain, medium chain, or long chain; whereas mono- and polyunsaturated fats are all long chain. MCT oil is a type of saturated fat that is shorter in length than other saturated fats. Although MCT is a saturated fat, it is not believed to increase the risk of coronary heart disease as with other saturated fats.

MCT oil is not believed to affect total cholesterol. However, it does cause a small increase in triglycerides. It has 10 percent fewer calories than long-chain triglycerides (LCTs) such as olive oil, avocados, and nuts. MCT oil can produce ketones, which are made from the breakdown of fat on low-carbohydrate diets. It can help you stay in a fat-burning state known as ketosis. This can increase the fat-burning benefits of intermittent fasting or following a low carbohydrate diet. Since intermittent fasting can have benefits for midlife women in regulating blood glucose and insulin levels, MCT oil can be a good addition to the diet.

MCT oil may also help optimize the growth of good bacteria and support the gut lining. Women approaching menopause tend to have a compromised gut microbiome. MCT oil can be helpful for maintaining a proper balance of bacteria. MCT oil also has been shown to increase the production of two hormones that aid satiety and fullness, leptin and peptide YY. According to research, this may result in weight loss because less food is being consumed.

Start slow with MCT oil. I recommend a half teaspoon in the beginning. Consuming too much may cause bloating, cramping, gas, or diarrhea. It should not be used for cooking because it has a low smoke point. The research has been promising on MCT oil. However, more studies need to be done. Consult with your dietician or medical care provider to see if MCT oil may be something to consider. The MCT oil product I use is Simply Energy by Cynthia Thurlow.

Berberine

According to hundreds of studies, berberine helps lower blood glucose (sugar), which can potentially stimulate weight loss. It has been shown to be as effective as the drug metformin for reducing blood sugar in people with type 2 diabetes. Since many midlife women struggle with blood glucose dysregulation and insulin resistance, this can be a helpful supplement to include.

It can potentially do the following:

- Decrease insulin resistance
- Decrease sugar production in the liver
- Increase the beneficial bacteria in the gut
- Help with weight loss

> *Berberine can be a powerful supplement, and everyone responds differently to it. Some individuals taking berberine may find that their blood sugar levels dip too low at night. Be sure to discuss this supplement with your healthcare provider, particularly if you are taking prescription medications.*

Optimal GI and GI Detox

The products Optimal GI and GI Detox can possibly be beneficial if you struggle with digestive problems. These products contain a variety of ingredients designed to do the following:

- Create healthy tissues in the gastrointestinal tract
- Normalize and regulate bowel movements
- Provide digestive comfort
- Normalize detoxification pathways

Eliminating toxic overload and buildup is important. Otherwise, the toxins will be recirculated back through organs, especially through the liver. Toxins have the potential to injure the body's cells and tissues. When a toxic burden increases, it is stored in fat cells, resulting in an increase in fat cells and even weight-loss resistance. As you lose weight, the fat cells shrink and the toxins are released into the body. If toxins are not removed from the body, they are scooped up and placed back into the fat cells.

I had a client who was exposed to mold. She gained weight and had difficulty losing the weight until she worked with a doctor who specialized in exposure to mold. The doctor explained that the weight gain was her body's way of protecting her from the toxic overload.

Thankfully, our bodies are good at detoxifying. The problem occurs when the exposure is more than our bodies can handle. This is especially true in our modern society where we are exposed to additives, chemicals, pollutants, cleaning products, and our self-care products, such as makeup and lotions. We may need to provide our bodies with extra help. Here are the two products I prefer:

- Optimal GI by Full Script (You will need a practitioner to subscribe this for you.)
- GI Detox by Biocidin

Digestive Enzymes

The body requires digestive enzymes to break down a meal. However, there may not be enough due to age, lifestyle, an inherited genetic deficiency (like lactose intolerance), or even overindulgence. Partially undigested food leads to fermentation in the gut, resulting in bloating, gas, indigestion, and constipation or diarrhea. As women move toward menopause, they are more vulnerable to digestive issues because of an imbalance of the gut microbiome. Supplementing with digestive enzymes can help with digestion. They can also increase energy and absorption of nutrients.

Adaptogenic Herbs

Adaptogenic herbs work to counteract the effects of stress in the body. As we've looked at in several chapters in this book already, over time stress can potentially harm the neurological, endocrine, digestive, and immune systems. Adaptogens have properties that can help to counteract harmful effects in the body due to stress. Adaptogens work at a molecular level by stabilizing the balance in the hypothalamic, pituitary, and adrenal glands, which are involved in the stress response.

Adaptogens have been studied in both animals and isolated neuronal cells and found to have several positive effects on the body, such as:

- Neuroprotective elements for the brain. They may increase brain chemicals such as nerve growth factor and improve cognition and memory.
- Anti-fatigue properties
- Antidepressant effects
- Central nervous system stimulation, which increases our ability to deal with stress and improves cognition

MACA

MACA root is a Peruvian plant that grows in the Andes mountains. It is a cruciferous vegetable related to broccoli, cabbage, and kale. It has been associated with several potential benefits, including increasing libido, stamina, energy, mood, and metabolism, all of which can suffer during perimenopause, menopause, and post-menopause due to the changing hormones. It may reduce blood pressure and reduce menopausal symptoms. My favorite brand is Mighty Maca by Dr. Anna Cabeca.

Collagen Peptides

Collagen comprises approximately 30 percent of our body's protein. It supports skin elasticity, bones, muscles, joints, the lining of the digestive tract, and connective tissue. It also helps with blood vessels (by helping your blood to clot) and provides a protective cover for organs in the body. We produce less collagen as we age, and the existing collagen breaks down at a faster rate. In addition, factors such as autoimmune disease, ultraviolet light exposure, smoking, sugar intake, and refined carbs cause collagen to become weak and brittle.

Women experience a significant decrease in collagen after menopause. Everyone experiences a rapid decline after age 60. Considering that we lose skin elasticity, muscle mass, and bone density once we cross the threshold of menopause, it can potentially be beneficial to supplement with collagen.

Creatine

Creatine is an amino acid located mostly in the muscles and the brain. It can be found in seafood and red meat. It's important for muscle synthesis and athletic performance. Creatine has also been used to improve brain health and cognition. Creatine is one of the most researched supplements on the market. Until recently, it was only marketed to men in the bodybuilding community. Recently, the benefits for women have emerged. Most women do not have enough creatine. Supplementation for midlife women is beneficial for several reasons:

- Muscle growth—when we transition to menopause, we begin losing muscle at up to 10 percent per decade.

- Cognition—when we lose estrogen, we are more vulnerable to cognitive and memory problems.
- Skin aging—it is believed that creatine can reduce wrinkles (particularly in the cream form).
- Prevention of injury to bones, muscles, ligaments, tendons, and nerves—as we age, we become far more prone to injury.
- Bone density—as women, we are at a higher risk of osteoporosis once we are in menopause.

The recommended dose for women is 2.5 to 3 grams per day. I combine mine with my collagen and protein powder. My favorite brands are 1st Phorm and Cynthia Thurlow.

There are many more supplements I could recommend. However, these are the ones which I consider to be more beneficial for women in midlife and beyond. While not every supplement is exclusively for women in perimenopause and menopause, each one can help to improve the overall results we are trying to achieve with our health and fitness goals at this unique stage of life.

In the next chapter, I will be addressing one of the number one questions I receive from women. Women often ask if I use hormone replacement therapy (HRT) or if recommend it for menopausal women. While I cannot say if this is the right choice for you, I can give you the facts as I understand them. With this knowledge, you can have an open discussion with your doctor about HRT and whether it's right for you.

Chapter 9

Is Hormone Replacement Therapy Right for Every Woman?

Having worked with over a thousand women in my coaching career, I have seen the effects of hormone replacement therapy on cognition, alleviation of menopausal symptoms, libido, and energy level.

Heather joined my Fit and Fierce coaching program with a goal of weight loss. She was 51 years old and was plagued by an extra 20 pounds she wanted to lose. As I had more discussions with Heather, I realized that some of her weight gain could potentially be related to lack of motivation. As she told me, "I lost my mojo. I don't care about anything anymore." She went on to tell me that she didn't really understand why she felt this way. She had a loving family and a career she enjoyed. There was no history of depression. In fact, these symptoms seemed to come out of nowhere.

Since Heather was transitioning into menopause, I suggested that she have hormone testing done. I gave her a referral to see my nurse practitioner, and she followed through with the testing. The results showed that her testosterone was almost at *zero. Other hormones were low as well. However, testosterone is often associated with motivation, confidence, and energy. Heather went on to have bio-identical hormone therapy. Within a few months, her mood improved and she began to lose weight. Today, Heather is at a healthy weight and enjoys regularly lifting weights. Her body composition has greatly improved (less body fat and more muscle).*

Knowing how to transition through menopause is a relatively new problem. For a white woman in the year 1900, the average life expectancy was 48.7 years. An African American woman's lifespan was only 33.5 years. Many women did not live long enough to experience menopause or all the changes to their bodies. Today, the average lifespan for a woman in the United States is 81 years. Not only does she experience menopause, but she lives on an additional three decades. On the surface, this may seem positive. It definitely is a better existence than how we lived over 120 years ago. However, life span is not the same as healthspan. In many cases the quality of a woman's life is low in those senior years. She is at risk for osteoporosis, cardiovascular disease, and cognitive decline such as dementia. According to Dr. Gabrelle Lyons, if a 65-year-old woman falls, she stands a 50 percent chance she will never walk again. Many times this is the result of losing skeletal muscle and bone density. The loss of the protection of estrogen plays a role in both.

When I was 48 years old, I went to lunch with a group of women from my spin class. At this point, I was experiencing perimenopausal symptoms but was in denial. Certainly, this was not happening to me. I remember the subject of hormone replacement therapy (HRT) came up in the conversation.

HRT is a medication or cream that contains hormones. It's taken primarily to replace the loss of estrogen, progesterone, and testosterone that occurs with menopause. It is used to reduce the symptoms of menopause, such as hot flashes, low libido, vaginal dryness, and bone loss.

One of the women was 67 years old and shared that she was using hormone replacement therapy. I was absolutely shocked. First, I didn't think a woman that age needed HRT. (I was underestimating the severity of menopausal symptoms, something I'd come to realize once I experienced them myself.) Second, the idea of hormones terrified me. I told her I would never use them.

I will never forget what she said in that moment. She looked me in the eye and said, "When you can't sleep, your sex life is gone, and you want to chase your husband with a butcher knife, you WILL change your mind." I was horrified. I left lunch certain I would never do hormone replacement therapy, no matter what happened to my body.

Three years later, I was 51 years old and training with my first bodybuilding coach for my second competition. I was struggling with sleep, night sweats, and hot flashes. My hair was thinning, and I wasn't building muscle despite the hours I was spending in the gym. My coach suggested I see her nurse practitioner who specializes in hormones. I reluctantly agreed.

I nervously walked into Melissa's office for the first time. She was kind, knowledgeable, and thorough. She asked me several questions about libido, sleep, energy, and nutrition. At this point, my nutrition was on point. However, sleep, libido, and energy were not. After extensive testing, the results showed high cortisol and virtually no estrogen and progesterone. My testosterone was completely tanked.

Melissa prescribed bio-identical estrogen, progesterone, and testosterone creams along with a DHEA supplement.

"Bio-identical" hormones simply mean that they are close to what your body would naturally produce. (We return to this later in the chapter.) This marked the beginning of my experience with hormone replacement therapy and the beginning of a long relationship with Melissa, who remains my practitioner 10 years later.

I can still recall how frightened I was to use hormone replacement. There was a reason for my fear. There's an infamous US study known as the Women's Health Initiative (WHI) that followed 16,000 women and spanned nine years that was published in 2002. The news was grim for women. This study caused widespread fear and changed the trajectory of treatment for women who had transitioned through menopause. Twenty years later, many women are still in fear.

The study reported that menopausal women taking estrogen and progesterone therapy were more likely to develop breast cancer, heart disease, stroke, and blood clots. As a result, many women stopped taking hormone therapy.

It was later revealed that there were major flaws in the study. Two-thirds of the women were 12 to 15 years past the onset of menopause, over 60 years old. The average age was 62.7. Only 10 percent were in their fifties. The remainder were in their seventies. Some were as old as 79. Because of age, the women over 60 were at an increased risk of heart disease, stroke, and breast cancer. There were a significant number of women who dropped out of the study. The majority of the women were overweight.

Seventy percent of the women in the study were over the age of 60 and took only one type of HRT, Prempro. Prempro is a pill combining synthetic progesterone and estrogen made from horse's urine. Synthetic hormones have been associated with cancer. In addition, the dose is believed to have been too high for the older women. In 2011 and 2012, women who received only the synthetic estrogen and no synthetic progesterone had fewer deaths each year for 10 years and were less likely to develop breast cancer and heart disease compared to those who received the placebo.

In addition, the increased breast cancer risk was much less than initially reported and amounted to four extra cases per 1,000 women after five years. This risk is actually lower than the risk associated with smoking, drinking alcohol, and obesity.

Many researchers and doctors have now come forward stating that the study actually harmed women who would have benefited from bio-identical therapy. Twenty years later, we are seeing the consequences for women. In the 2019 paper "The Controversial History of Hormone Replacement Therapy," researchers Angelo Cagnacci and Martina Venier report, "HRT use and its consolidation by the publication of the WHI trial, which was inadequately designed, evaluated, and reported. The damage done was huge, basically leaving many symptomatic women without an effective treatment."

We continue to see the consequences of this 20-year-old study, including a surge in osteoporosis. During and after menopause, when we lose estrogen, we lose the protection for our brain, muscles, bones, and heart. Loss of muscle leads to weakness and excess adipose (body fat) tissue. Lack of estrogen sacrifices bone density. A loss of bone density can result in a condition called osteoporosis. Osteoporosis causes bones to become so weak and brittle that even coughing could cause a fracture.

Cognition is also at risk. At the very least, women suffer brain fog in the perimenopausal to menopausal years. The role of estrogen in brain health is being heavily researched. It is believed that the estrogen deficit is one of the reasons women experience a higher risk for dementia and Alzheimer's disease. However, no definitive conclusions have been made, and further studies are needed.

Progesterone, which we've discussed earlier in the book, is a hormone we often overlook. Sleep disruption and anxiety are also factors in menopause. Progesterone aids with both mood and sleep and works in balance with estrogen.

When I first walked through Melissa's door, the study was 10 years old and was already drawing criticism. After years of hearing frightening news stories and having my doctor discourage the use of hormones, I could not quiet my fears. However, I instantly trusted Melissa who calmed my concerns, and I reluctantly agreed to try HRT.

Within a few months, my life changed for the better. I started to put on muscle. My skin and hair improved. The night sweats and hot flashes were gone. My libido was back. The brain fog lifted. I did not realize how much I'd been suffering until I felt like Carol again.

Women who enter early menopause can benefit from HRT. A 2012 analysis reported that women who started HRT within 10 years of menopause had a 30 percent lower mortality rate and a 48 percent lower risk of heart disease than those taking a placebo.

The biggest takeaway from this study is that many doctors are still basing their treatment recommendations on a 20-year-old, heavily flawed study. It's important to note that there is an entire generation of general practitioners, endocrinologists, and gynecologists, who are afraid to prescribe HRT. Because of a faulty study, they have been left without the confidence or the knowledge to do so. Thus, it is important to choose a practitioner with the experience to help a woman navigate through this important transition of life.

I do not believe every woman should do HRT. Women should carefully weigh the benefits and any risks and discuss the options with their doctor. However, women need to be informed with facts before they make a decision as to whether or not HRT is an option for them. Knowledge is empowering and the only way to make the best decision possible.

HRT alone will not result in the changes a woman wants to see and feel. It's important to address all the lifestyle pieces from nutrition and exercise to sleep and stress. When I sought help from Melissa, I had already implemented significant changes in my nutrition and exercise. However, HRT greatly improved my quality of life and made my lifestyle changes even more effective.

Let's discuss bio-identical hormones further. As mentioned, "bio-identical" hormones simply mean that they are close to what your body would naturally produce. Prescriptions for estradiol patches or vaginal suppositories are not labeled as bio-identical. However, they are bio-identical because they are estradiol, the main form of estrogen produced in a woman's body. Compounded bio-identical hormones are made by a compounding pharmacist from a medical provider's prescription. They come in the form of creams, injectables, implants, suppositories, and oral sublingual tablets. They are not regulated and can have variances in the formulas, which are not always true to the label. I personally use a combination of compounded formulas and hormones covered by insurance. It's best not to assume that all compounded formulas are "healthier," more natural options. Ultimately, that can be a marketing ploy. Women should be well informed consumers and CEOs of their own bodies. As mentioned, work in alliance with an experienced medical practitioner to determine the best solution.

I often receive messages from males interested in my health and body coaching who ask, "What about us?" Yes, men do go through andropause later in life. However, men go through far fewer hormonal shifts in their lifetime than do women. They move from prepuberty to puberty and into adulthood. They also do not lose their reproductive capabilities. Men continue to produce sperm even after they die! For days after they die, they continue to produce sperm. They continue to make testosterone as well. In men, testosterone is converted into estrogen in the brain and is the primary source of estrogen for the male brain. Both men and women convert testosterone to estrogen. However, older men produce more than menopausal women. The average male at age 60 has four times the amount of estrogen in his body and brain as the average woman at age 60 not doing HRT. Men get less osteoporosis and dementia than women.

The decision to do HRT is a woman's choice. I know women who never did hormone replacement therapy and transitioned smoothly into menopause. However, the benefits for cognition and bone health are important considerations. A woman should never make this decision based on fear or a study which was severely flawed. Rather, she should decide based on the facts and after careful consideration with her healthcare provider. If her provider does not want to have the discussion, I believe in finding another practitioner.

As we move into the final chapter, I want you to consider what you would like your life to be after menopause. After all, life is not over. In fact, it can be a new beginning. I did not contemplate this part of my life. In my forties, I was so busy with my children, aging parents, and —eventually—reentry into the workforce that I never took the time to think about how my life would look in my fifties, sixties, and beyond. Looking back, I believe I was fearful of aging. My friend, I do not want you to have fear. I want you to see the possibilities of the future.

Chapter 10

Seeing the Possibilities

Women in midlife—in perimenopause, menopause, and post-menopause—can feel particularly vulnerable to feelings of abandonment. Menopause is the most challenging transition most women will encounter next to puberty. Perimenopause is referred to as reverse puberty. It's a time where a woman can feel confused or alone. When midlife women feel abandoned by their doctors and society, they start to give up on themselves and the possibilities ahead. It's common for a woman to feel like she doesn't belong after she goes through menopause. Depression can seep into the very soul, and even cognitive ability can decline. It's a time women need to ask themselves and other women the questions:

- What is my/your story?
- What scares me/you the most?
- What brings me/you joy?
- How can I/you give and seek support?
- What do I/you want to accomplish in my/your transition into this stage of life?

I did not ask myself the questions. I was swept up into my fifties after decades of marriage, children, and careers. When we are swept into menopause, everything can feel like a blur. We can feel a tug on the mind to fulfill a long-forgotten or even unknown desire. My family and my faith are the absolute highlight and foundation of my life. Yet, I felt there was an unfinished purpose that I needed to fulfill. For me, I needed to work through what was unresolved from my past in order to help others and to be the strong woman I know I was meant to be.

Recently I recorded an episode of the *Forever Fit with Carol Covino* podcast on the psychology of aging. I shared my fears and what I was changing in my life at the age of 61. My fifties were all about improving physically. As I turned 60, my focus shifted from the outward to the inward. I wanted a deeper connection in my marriage and my faith. I wanted to enjoy every moment with my now adult kids. When I recorded the episode, I felt vulnerable. I shared a fear of death I had literally not spoken aloud to anyone. I didn't know how the episode would be received by women. Yet many messaged me to say that I had said the very things they were thinking. They shared their fears with me, just as I had with them. In doing so, the fears seemed not as daunting.

Women in menopause are a powerful group. Our needs and desires matter. Your needs and desires matter. We should not be expected to abandon our vitality, suffer through endless sleepless nights, or go through our days in a fog. Life is not over. Menopause is a normal passage in life and should be celebrated rather than feared. As women, we need to cast away shame.

There are wonderful benefits to this stage of life:

- A decrease in estrogen changes the way the menopausal woman handles anger. As a young woman, she tended to stifle any urge to stand up for herself. Estrogen is the "people-pleasing" hormone. As estrogen levels decrease, her need to speak up for what she believes to be right becomes stronger, which is incredibly empowering and satisfying.

- Because the menopausal woman is no longer tied to a hormonal cycle, she is free to find her purpose from within rather than externally. She is able to lean into her own wisdom and experience.

- She is more focused and doesn't feel the need to do 20 things at once. Time is precious, and she wants to fill her time with the people and things that matter.

Just yesterday, my husband and I took a long hike from the base of the Sandia Mountains to the crest. We recently rediscovered the joy of hiking, something we had not fully done since having kids. The hike seemed pretty straightforward. We would take a familiar trail up to a fork in the path known as the T. From there we would hike the crest trail to the restaurant and tram at the top. We would have lunch and take the tram down. The hike was 7.5 to 8 miles long and mostly an uphill climb.

Well, let's just say things did not go as planned. We made it to the T and turned on to the crest. From there, the trails were poorly marked if at all. At one juncture we apparently made a wrong turn and hiked an additional three miles in the wrong direction. The forest was thick. We weren't seeing any other hikers and the afternoon was slipping away. I'd had a premonition when we initially took the path. It just hadn't felt right to me. I told my husband who assured me I was wrong, yet I couldn't shake the feeling.

As we walked, I thought of all the possibilities. Maybe we were on the right path and would see the tram behind the next corner. Perhaps we should turn around and go back down the mountain on the same path we had taken up. I looked at my watch and realized part of that hike would be past nightfall. If we continued walking in the wrong direction, we'd have to spend the night in the mountains.

Thankfully, my worst fears were not a reality. We ran into one sole hiker who happened to know the trails very well. He escorted us back to where the trailhead split into three different paths. Sure enough, we had missed a turn. He pointed us in the correct direction and went on his way. There were still an additional two-plus miles we needed to travel to reach the tram. The path was steep with switchbacks, and at times I worried we had once again missed a turn. Relief flooded us both when we heard the tram cables and eventually saw the steep steps leading up to the lookout and the restaurant.

The hike brought several things to my mind. First and foremost, I was thankful to God for sending the lone hiker to our rescue. Secondly, I thought about how often we give up before we reach the top. Third, I meditated on all the things that can set us back. We can take the wrong path. At times we can feel lost and scared. Branches and thick brush tear at our arms and legs. There are large boulders and rocks we can trip on and fall if we're not careful. Clouds roll in, and thunder is on the horizon.

The similarities between our life transitions and my hike seemed very much the same to me. The early forties lead us into the confusion of perimenopause. Are we doing the right things to support our body or are we going in the wrong direction? At times we feel battered, just like I did when branches tore my skin to blood. As we move toward menopause, we may feel time is running out, and we're headed toward the cold darkness. We experience overwhelming anxiety and fear as well as fatigue due to the night sweats, hot flashes, and sleep and energy disturbances.

Then there is the hope we see in the distance if we don't allow our minds to take us further off the path. Our mindset and how we care for our body is what will determine if we make it to the top and enjoy the sunset or if we remain lost on the trails. Ultimately, it's our mindset that determines this path. Nothing happens with our nutrition, exercise, and lifestyle without our willingness to embrace a new stage of life. That comes down to making a decision—to embrace it or not. Deciding to find passion and purpose, having gratitude, and dealing with past trauma and regrets with self-compassion determine whether or not we age with vitality.

As we conclude this journey, I want to invite you to reach out to me and to be a part of my community. I would love to hear your thoughts and know your story. I am always available for questions. There are several ways to connect. You can listen to my podcast, *Forever Fit with Carol Covino*. You can send me a message on Instagram @carolcovinofitness. You can also find me on YouTube (@carolcovinofitness). If you would like to explore working with me in the future, consider joining my next round of the 12-week Fit and Fierce program for women over 40. You can find the program details on my website, https//carolcovino.com, or email me at carol@carolcovino.com. I look forward to hearing from you!

References

Chapter 1

Antoni, R., Robertson, T., Robertson, M., & Johnston, J. (2018). A pilot feasibility study exploring the effects of a moderate time-restricted feeding intervention on energy intake, adiposity and metabolic physiology in free-living human subjects. *Journal of Nutritional Science, 7*, E22. doi:10.1017/jns.2018.13

Cabeca, A. (2019). *The Hormone Fix: Burn Fat Naturally, Boost Energy, Sleep Better, and Stop Hot Flashes, the Keto-Green Way.* Ballantine Books.

Collins, B. C., Laakkonen, E. K., & Lowe, D. A. (2019). Aging of the musculoskeletal system: How the loss of estrogen impacts muscle strength. *Bone, 123*, 137–144. https://doi.org/10.1016/j.bone.2019.03.033

Galgani, J. E., Moro, C., & Ravussin, E. (2008). Metabolic flexibility and insulin resistance. *American Journal of Physiology – Endocrinology and Metabolism, 295*(5), E1009–E1017. https://doi.org/10.1152/ajpendo.90558.2008

Golbidi, S., Daiber, A., Korac, B., Li, H., Essop, M. F., & Laher, I. (2017). Health Benefits of Fasting and Caloric Restriction. *Current Diabetes Reports*, *17*(12), 123. https://doi.org/10.1007/s11892-017-0951-7

Goodpaster, B. H., & Sparks, L. M. (2017). Metabolic Flexibility in Health and Disease. *Cell Metabolism*, *25*(5), 1027–1036. https://doi.org/10.1016/j.cmet.2017.04.015

Chapter 2

Deol, P., Kozlova, E., Valdez, M., Ho, C., Yang, E. W., Richardson, H., Gonzalez, G., Truong, E., Reid, J., Valdez, J., Deans, J. R., Martinez-Lomeli, J., Evans, J. R., Jiang, T., Sladek, F. M., & Curras-Collazo, M. C. (2020). Dysregulation of Hypothalamic Gene Expression and the Oxytocinergic System by Soybean Oil Diets in Male Mice. *Endocrinology*, *161*(2). https://doi.org/10.1210/endocr/bqz044

Gower, B. A., & Goss, A. M. (2015). A lower-carbohydrate, higher-fat diet reduces abdominal and intermuscular fat and increases insulin sensitivity in adults at risk of type 2 diabetes. *The Journal of Nutrition*, *145*(1), 177S–83S. https://doi.org/10.3945/jn.114.195065

Shanahan, C. (2020) *The Fatburn Fix: Boost Energy, End Hunger, and Lose Weight by Using Body Fat for Fuel.* New York, NY: Flatiron Books.

University of California - Riverside. (2020, January 17). America's most widely consumed oil causes genetic changes in the brain: Soybean oil linked to metabolic and neurological changes in mice. *ScienceDaily*.

Retrieved October 14, 2022 from www.sciencedaily.com/releases/2020/01/200117080827.htm

Virgin, J.J. (2013) *The Virgin Diet: Drop 7 Foods, Lose 7 Pounds, Just 7 Days*. New York, NY: Harlequin.

Chapter 3

Bellisle, F., McDevitt, R., & Prentice, A. M. (1997). Meal frequency and energy balance. *The British Journal of Nutrition*, *77 Suppl 1*, S57–S70. https://doi.org/10.1079/bjn19970104

Blasbalg, T. L., Hibbeln, J. R., Ramsden, C. E., Majchrzak, S. F., & Rawlings, R. R. (2011). Changes in consumption of omega-3 and omega-6 fatty acids in the United States during the 20th century. *The American Journal of Clinical Nutrition*, *93*(5), 950–962. https://doi.org/10.3945/ajcn.110.006643

Cameron, J. D., Cyr, M. J., & Doucet, E. (2010). Increased meal frequency does not promote greater weight loss in subjects who were prescribed an 8-week equi-energetic energy-restricted diet. *The British Journal of Nutrition*, *103*(8), 1098–1101. https://doi.org/10.1017/S0007114509992984

Igwe, O., Sone, M., Matveychuk, D., Baker, G. B., & Dursun, S. M. (2021). A review of effects of calorie restriction and fasting with potential relevance to depression. *Progress in Neuro-Osychopharmacology & Biological Psychiatry*, *111*, 110206. https://doi.org/10.1016/j.pnpbp.2020.110206

Kim, M. K., Han, K., Park, Y. M., Kwon, H. S., Kang, G., Yoon, K. H., & Lee, S. H. (2018). Associations of Variability in Blood Pressure, Glucose and Cholesterol Concentrations, and Body Mass Index With Mortality and Cardiovascular Outcomes in the General Population. *Circulation*, *138*(23), 2627–2637. https://doi.org/10.1161/CIRCULATIONAHA.118.034978

Li, G., Xie, C., Lu, S., Nichols, R. G., Tian, Y., Li, L., Patel, D., Ma, Y., Brocker, C. N., Yan, T., Krausz, K. W., Xiang, R., Gavrilova, O., Patterson, A. D., & Gonzalez, F. J. (2017). Intermittent Fasting Promotes White Adipose Browning and Decreases Obesity by Shaping the Gut Microbiota. *Cell Metabolism*, *26*(4), 672–685. e4. https://doi.org/10.1016/j.cmet.2017.08.019

Thurlow, C. (2022) *Intermittent Fasting Transformation: The 45-Day Program for Women to Lose Stubborn Weight, Improve Hormonal Health, and Slow Aging*. New York: Avery.

Chapter 4

Cadegiani, F. A., & Kater, C. E. (2017). Hypothalamic-Pituitary-Adrenal (HPA) Axis Functioning in Overtraining Syndrome: Findings from Endocrine and Metabolic Responses on Overtraining Syndrome (EROS)-EROS-HPA Axis. *Sports Medicine - Open*, *3*(1), 45. https://doi.org/10.1186/s40798-017-0113-0

Fisher, G., McCarthy, J. P., Zuckerman, P. A., Bryan, D. R., Bickel, C. S., & Hunter, G. R. (2013). Frequency of combined resistance and aerobic training in older women. *Journal of Strength and Conditioning Research, 27*(7), 1868–1876. https://doi.org/10.1519/JSC.0b013e31827367e0

Hunter, G. R., Bickel, C. S., Fisher, G., Neumeier, W. H., & McCarthy, J. P. (2013). Combined aerobic and strength training and energy expenditure in older women. *Medicine and Science in Sports and Exercise, 45*(7), 1386–1393. https://doi.org/10.1249/MSS.0b013e3182860099

Ko, J., & Park, Y. M. (2021). Menopause and the Loss of Skeletal Muscle Mass in Women. *Iranian Journal of Public Health, 50*(2), 413–414. https://doi.org/10.18502/ijph.v50i2.5362

Kullmann, S., Goj, T., Veit, R., Fritsche, L., Wagner, L., Schneeweiss, P., Hoene, M., Hoffmann, C., Machann, J., Niess, A., Preissl, H., Birkenfeld, A. L., Peter, A., Häring, H. U., Fritsche, A., Moller, A., Weigert, C., & Heni, M. (2022). Exercise restores brain insulin sensitivity in sedentary adults who are overweight and obese. *JCI Insight, 7*(18), e161498. https://doi.org/10.1172/jci.insight.161498

Lee, D. H., Rezende, L., Joh, H. K., Keum, N., Ferrari, G., Rey-Lopez, J. P., Rimm, E. B., Tabung, F. K., & Giovannucci, E. L. (2022). Long-Term Leisure-Time Physical Activity Intensity and All-Cause and Cause-Specific Mortality: A Prospective Cohort of US Adults. *Circulation, 146*(7), 523–534. https://doi.org/10.1161/CIRCULATIONAHA.121.058162

Mishra, N., Mishra, V. N., & Devanshi (2011). Exercise beyond menopause: Dos and Don'ts. *Journal of Mid-Life Health, 2*(2), 51–56. https://doi.org/10.4103/0976-7800.92524

Tessier, A. J., Wing, S. S., Rahme, E., Morais, J. A., & Chevalier, S. (2022). Association of Low Muscle Mass With Cognitive Function During a 3-Year Follow-up Among Adults Aged 65 to 86 Years in the Canadian Longitudinal Study on Aging. *JAMA Network Open*, 5(7), e2219926. https://doi.org/10.1001/jamanetworkopen.2022.19926

Woods, R., Hess, R., Biddington, C., & Federico, M. (2020). Association of lean body mass to menopausal symptoms: The Study of Women's Health Across the Nation. *Women's Midlife Health*, 6, 10. https://doi.org/10.1186/s40695-020-00058-9

Chapter 5

Adverse Childhood Experiences. (2022). National Conference of State Legislatures. Retrieved October 15, 2022, from https://www.ncsl.org/research/health/adverse-childhood-experiences-aces.aspx

Apigian, A. (2022, August 7) *The Beginning of a Trauma Body, Trauma Healing Accelerated*. Retrieved October 15, 2022, from https://www.traumahealingaccelerated.com/the-beginning-of-a-trauma-body/

Mate, G. (2011) *When the Body Says No: Understanding the Stress-Disease Connection*. Hoboken, NJ: John Wiley & Sons.

Rosenheck R. (1986). Impact of posttraumatic stress disorder of World War II on the next generation. *The Journal of Nervous and Mental Disease*, 174(6), 319–327. https://doi.org/10.1097/00005053-198606000-00001

Scaer, R.C. (2001) *The Body Bears the Burden: Trauma, Dissociation, and Disease.* New York, NY: Haworth Medical Press.

Thurston, R. C., & Miller, E. (2019). Association of Interpersonal Violence With Women's Health. *JAMA Internal Medicine, 179*(1), 87–89. https://doi.org/10.1001/jamainternmed.2018.5242

Van der Kolk, B. (2015) *The Body Keeps the Score: Brain, Mind, and Body in the Healing of Trauma.* New York, NY: Penguin.

Van der Kolk, B., McFarlane, A.C. and Weisæth, L. (2007) *Traumatic Stress: The Effects of Overwhelming Experience on Mind, Body, and Society.* New York, NY: Guilford Press.

Verma, R., Balhara, Y. P., & Gupta, C. S. (2011). Gender differences in stress response: Role of developmental and biological determinants. *Industrial Psychiatry Journal, 20*(1), 4–10. https://doi.org/10.4103/0972-6748.98407

Chapter 6

Adams, J. W., Alosco, M. L., Mez, J., Alvarez, V. E., Huber, B. R., Tripodis, Y., Adler, C. H., Kubilius, C., Cormier, K. A., Mathais, R., Nicks, R., Kelley, H. J., Saltiel, N., Uretsky, M., Nair, E., Aytan, N., Cherry, J. D., Nowinski, C. J., Kowall, N. W., Goldstein, L. E., Stein, T. D. (2020). Association of probable REM sleep behavior disorder with pathology and years of contact sports play in chronic traumatic encephalopathy. *Acta Neuropathologica, 140*(6), 851–862. https://doi.org/10.1007/s00401-020-02206-x

Baumgartner, F. (2012, March 6). *The Capsule - Red Bull Stratos 2012*. YouTube. Retrieved October 15, 2022, from https://www.youtube.com/watch?v=se_1i9D3nYc

Bhaskar, S., Hemavathy, D., & Prasad, S. (2016). Prevalence of chronic insomnia in adult patients and its correlation with medical comorbidities. *Journal of Family Medicine and Primary Care*, 5(4), 780–784. https://doi.org/10.4103/2249-4863.201153

Crew, B. (2015, November 16) *Watch: Here's what happened when a teenager stayed awake for 11 Days straight, ScienceAlert*. Retrieved October 15, 2022, from https://www.sciencealert.com/watch-here-s-what-happened-when-a-teenager-stayed-awake-for-11-days-straight

Galgani, J. E., Moro, C., & Ravussin, E. (2008). Metabolic flexibility and insulin resistance. *American Journal of Physiology – Endocrinology and Metabolism*, 295(5), E1009–E1017. https://doi.org/10.1152/ajpendo.90558.2008

Izawa et al. (2019, September 20) *The brain may actively forget during dream sleep, National Institutes of Health*. U.S. Department of Health and Human Services. Retrieved October 15, 2022, from https://www.nih.gov/news-events/news-releases/brain-may-actively-forget-during-dream-sleep

Jawaid, A., Roszkowski, M., & Mansuy, I. M. (2018). Transgenerational Epigenetics of Traumatic Stress. *Progress in Molecular Biology and Translational Science, 158*, 273–298. https://doi.org/10.1016/bs.pmbts.2018.03.003

Jehan, S., Jean-Louis, G., Zizi, F., Auguste, E., Pandi-Perumal, S. R., Gupta, R., Attarian, H., McFarlane, S. I., Hardeland, R., & Brzezinski, A. (2017). Sleep, Melatonin, and the Menopausal Transition: What Are the Links? *Sleep Science (Sao Paulo, Brazil)*, *10*(1), 11–18. https://doi.org/10.5935/1984-0063.20170003

National Institute on Aging. (2020, November 12) *Sleep disturbances linked to abnormal deposits of certain proteins in the brain, U.S. Department of Health and Human Services*. Retrieved October 15, 2022, from https://www.nia.nih.gov/news/sleep-disturbances-linked-abnormal-deposits-certain-proteins-brain

Neckelmann, D., Mykletun, A., & Dahl, A. A. (2007). Chronic insomnia as a risk factor for developing anxiety and depression. *Sleep*, *30*(7), 873–880. https://doi.org/10.1093/sleep/30.7.873

Nutt, D., Wilson, S., & Paterson, L. (2008). Sleep disorders as core symptoms of depression. *Dialogues in Clinical Neuroscience*, *10*(3), 329–336. https://doi.org/10.31887/DCNS.2008.10.3/dnutt

Park, Y. S., Kim, S. H., Park, J. W., Kho, Y., Seok, P. R., Shin, J. H., Choi, Y. J., Jun, J. H., Jung, H. C., & Kim, E. K. (2020). Melatonin in the colon modulates intestinal microbiota in response to stress and sleep deprivation. *Intestinal Research*, *18*(3), 325–336. https://doi.org/10.5217/ir.2019.00093

Winer, J. R., Mander, B. A., Kumar, S., Reed, M., Baker, S. L., Jagust, W. J., & Walker, M. P. (2020). Sleep Disturbance Forecasts β-Amyloid Accumulation across Subsequent Years. *Current Biology*, *30*(21), 4291–4298.e3. https://doi.org/10.1016/j.cub.2020.08.017

Chapter 7

Collagen: What it is, Types, Function & Benefits. (n.d.). Cleveland Clinic. Retrieved October 15, 2022, from https://my.clevelandclinic. org/health/articles/23089-collagen

Kinsella, R., Maher, T., & Clegg, M. E. (2017). Coconut oil has less satiating properties than medium chain triglyceride oil. *Physiology & Behavior*, *179*, 422–426. https://doi.org/10.1016/j.physbeh.2017.07.007

Panossian, A., & Wikman, G. (2010). Effects of Adaptogens on the Central Nervous System and the Molecular Mechanisms Associated with Their Stress-Protective Activity. *Pharmaceuticals (Basel, Switzerland)*, *3*(1), 188–224. https://doi.org/10.3390/ph3010188

Ye, Y., Liu, X., Wu, N., Han, Y., Wang, J., Yu, Y., & Chen, Q. (2021). Efficacy and Safety of Berberine Alone for Several Metabolic Disorders: A Systematic Review and Meta-Analysis of Randomized Clinical Trials. *Frontiers in Pharmacology*, *12*, 653887. https://doi.org/10.3389/fphar.2021.653887

Chapter 8

Brizendine, L. (2022). *The Upgrade: How the Female Brain Gets Stronger and Better in Midlife and Beyond.* Hay House UK, London.

Cagnacci, A., & Venier, M. (2019). The Controversial History of Hormone Replacement Therapy. *Medicina (Kaunas, Lithuania)*, *55*(9), 602. https:// doi.org/10.3390/medicina55090602

Clark J. H. (2006). A critique of Women's Health Initiative Studies (2002-2006). *Nuclear Receptor Signaling, 4,* e023. https://doi.org/10.1621/nrs.04023

Manson, J. E., Aragaki, A. K., Rossouw, J. E., Anderson, G. L., Prentice, R. L., LaCroix, A. Z., Chlebowski, R. T., Howard, B. V., Thomson, C. A., Margolis, K. L., Lewis, C. E., Stefanick, M. L., Jackson, R. D., Johnson, K. C., Martin, L. W., Shumaker, S. A., Espeland, M. A., Wactawski-Wende, J., & WHI Investigators (2017). Menopausal Hormone Therapy and Long-term All-Cause and Cause-Specific Mortality: The Women's Health Initiative Randomized Trials. *JAMA, 318*(10), 927–938. https://doi.org/10.1001/jama.2017.11217

Robinson, L.; Medical Advisory Council of the British Menopause Society. (2020, November). HRT: Benefits and risks. Retrieved October 15, 2022, from https://www.womens-health-concern. org/wp-content/uploads/2021/01/11-WHC-FACTSHEET-HRT-BenefitsRisks-JAN2021-B.pdf

Thurlow. (2022, September 3). *The Upgrade: A Unique Perspective on Perimenopause and Menopause with Dr. Louann Brizendine* (episode 227). Retrieved October 15, 2022, from https://www. listennotes.com/podcasts/everyday-wellness/ ep-227-the-upgrade-a-unique-OtwmDCVkABu/ embed/

Acknowledgments

Writing this book has been a labor of love. None of this would have been possible without my faith and my family. There was a time several years ago when I never would have believed writing a book would have been possible. It was a time where I felt God was silent, and I had lost my faith. I learned that God never leaves or forsakes us. We just need to be still and listen. This is what I did and what has brought me to this place.

I am forever grateful to my husband, Mike, who is my best friend, my rock, and the love of my life. He believes in me even when I don't believe in myself. I would not be writing this book without him. He never fails to encourage me when I need it most, and he knows exactly what to say when I need it the most.

To my three children, who are my everything and whom I love more than life itself. We crossed oceans to bring home these three beautiful children. My daughter Francesca is my biggest cheerleader. We talked about this book during many lunch dates. My daughter Sophia is always in my corner and has the dearest heart. My son, Tony, is miles away serving in the Navy, yet he never fails to tell me how proud he is of me.

To all the women I have worked with over the years—you were my inspiration for writing this book. As I dove into each chapter, I saw your faces, felt your struggle, and rejoiced in your triumphs.

Finally, to the women who will read this book—it is my hope that you see the transition into menopause as something beautiful.

About the Author

Carol Covino is a health and fitness coach for women over 40 who are struggling with hormonal symptoms from perimenopause and menopause. She helps them to transition through this beautiful but challenging part of life and to reach their health goals through nutrition, exercise, and lifestyle habits. Carol is a certified menopause specialist. She also holds certifications in fitness nutrition, female metabolism, and personal training.

Carol is the creator of the Slim Stomach Solution and the Fit and Fierce program for women over 40. She also hosts the *Forever Fit with Carol Covino* podcast. She has been a guest speaker at many international virtual events, including the Biohacking Conference for Women.

Carol is a former national bikini bodybuilding champion and has competed in 15 shows. She is an avid weightlifter. When Carol is not coaching, she is spending time with her children and husband of 36 years. On Saturdays, you can find her with a weighted ruck pack hiking through the Sandia Mountains of New Mexico with her husband.

Printed in Great Britain
by Amazon

26192678R00121